like stanzas in a poem

Notes

Yoga at the Wall

for Beginning Students and
their Teachers

Nancy McCaochan

with Lynn Medow
photographs by Susann Spilkin

In the Company of Women
Royal Oak, Michigan

1700 Ferris Ave.
Royal Oak, MI 48067
www.in-the-company-of-women.com

Published in the USA, 2008

A NOTE TO THE READER:
The information regarding benefits of the various yoga postures and exercises presented
in this book has been gleaned from time-honored traditions of health maintenance and
is intended to supplement--not replace--recommendations from the medical community
and other health care professionals. Neither is it intended to be prescriptive regarding the
treatment of injury or illness. Rather it presents one approach to maintaining physical well-
being. As with any program of physical conditioning, readers should consult their physician
before beginning the practices described in this book. In addition, it should be noted that
contraindications for the poses are not inclusive, so readers are advised to continue to consult
regularly with their primary care providers, particularly if they experience any symptoms that
might require diagnosis or medical treatment. The author and publisher shall not
be liable for any loss, injury or damage allegedly incurred from the use of the information
provided in this book.

ISBN 978-0-615-22231-8

In the Company of Women was founded in
2003 to promote women's enterprises.
This is its first publication.

To Nancy Steen and Lois Miller, as promised so long ago.

Contents

Preface

Yoga first came to me with a boyfriend. I was 24 and Daniel, avidly reading Ram Das' *Be Here Now*, taught me the few poses that were included in the book. We practiced daily for the year we lived together in southern Mendocino County, California. Just before we split up, we visited a mutual friend. One of *his* friends amazed me. He had the most awesome posture I'd ever seen—military in bearing but relaxed and open at the same time. I asked him where he'd learned to do that.

"Yoga," was his answer.

He recommended *Light on Yoga*, by B. K. S. Iyengar, one of the pre-eminent yoga teachers of our time. I bought the book and began to study. I practiced daily and taught briefly for the recreation department in my hometown. In my mid-twenties, I was filled with restless energy and, without a social network that supported my yoga practice, I began to drift.

Disposed toward the mystical, I had a vision of Jesus, gave up yoga, got married, returned to Catholicism, raised a family. Then graduate school and an ensuing divorce left me reeling. I remembered that yoga had helped me feel centered. By this time, even in rural southeastern Ohio, where my husband was employed, people were interested in yoga. One of the most popular local teachers had studied with Mr. Iyengar and his children. I resumed my practice and began to explore other traditions—Kripalu, Sivananda, and Integral. In order to deepen my understanding and to overcome the inertia of non-practice, I began to teach.

Although I was able to find valuable insights about technique and philosophy from most of the sessions, I discovered that, given time alone on my mat, my first impulse was to surf the resistance in my body. I worked slowly and methodically, breathing into dense places until they became more spacious. From this work, an intuitive, tactile understanding of the movement of prana emerged. In addition, through experimentation and attention, the workings of muscles and bones and their relationships to one another became apparent. My resistances were my greatest teachers. I began to take poses apart, piece by resistant piece, working through stuck places only to find that others appeared. Once they, too, had yielded to breath and leverage, other constrictions surfaced, were opened, and replaced with still others in seeming endless succession. I came to understand two things. First, yoga is a process of unfolding. More importantly, yoga sharpens our minds so that we see ever more clearly—both how our bodies function and how our energies are configured.

For many of us, the real yoga begins when we leave the practice room. Moving our bodies in space, meeting with and going beyond the resistance we find in muscles and connective tissue—these are the tasks of hatha yoga. But the lessons of practice, of *sadhana*, can be extrapolated. Over time they work themselves into our social, emotional and professional lives. In a process of continual unfolding, we learn how to move slowly through and beyond a seeming obstacle while honoring the reason for its existence.

Most of us are bound up in profound ways. We're afraid to say what we feel, reluctant to try new things or too concerned about what "they" think. As a result, we build up emotional armoring that's reflected in our bodies as well as in the ways we work, play and interact with others. Yoga, at its best, disarms us.

Sometimes there's a lovely and beneficent insight that accompanies our physical *sadhana*, so that loosening the hips allows us to feel sensuality more deeply. Sometimes strengthening our core trims excess emotionality from our psyche. But sometimes nothing we do to our physical bodies seems to make any difference. No matter how long we hold ourselves in pigeon, we leave class with our psoas as tight as it was when we began our practice. Or our minds remain distracted despite the heat and intensity of the vinyasa flow.

At such times, we need a little help to liberate us from the intransigence of our patterns. We need another way of looking at the world. May this small book be such an aide. May it serve you in your yoga, a path to greater awareness, peace, and joy.

Introduction

Hatha yoga is the best-known of the 8 limbs of classical yoga, a comprehensive system of human development. The goal of the system is neither better muscular definition nor greater range of motion in the joints. Rather it's the elimination of individual suffering through the evolution of one's consciousness. To this end, moral practices and ethical observances combine with attention to physical well-being, breathing exercises and techniques for mental focus and concentration. The person who adheres faithfully to this regimen becomes progressively more free of many of the problems that besiege humankind—anxiety, hypertension, depression, anger, acute and/or chronic illness.

Some of us who show up regularly for practice were first attracted to yoga because we needed a good stretch to supplement our workout. Or we met someone who had extraordinary posture or an extraordinary light in their eyes, and we wanted to be like them. The health benefits of a regular yoga practice *are* wonderful: better respiration, decreased blood pressure, greater muscle tone and increased vitality. These, however, are all by-products of a system that noted yoga historian Georg Feuerstein, Ph.D. calls a "psychotechnology."

Yoga, one of the 6 schools of Hindu philosophy, has been practiced in India since antiquity. The *Sutras* of Patanjali are commonly considered the first written record of the practices. It's here that the 8-limbs are elaborated. Scholars differ about who Patanjali was and when he lived, placing him either in 200. B.CE or in 200 C.E. Regardless of the date, he is a seminal figure in the evolution of yoga. Legend has it that he was an incarnation of Ananta, the thousand-headed serpent upon whom the god Vishnu (who is responsible for sustaining all life) rode across the waters of the universe. The name Patanjali was given to him when he "fell from heaven" (*pata,* "falling") into the "cupped palms" (*anjali*) of a devout woman during her morning prayers. Thus yoga—the skillful means by which human beings can ride the currents of their lives—was brought to earth.

In the 2nd of the *Sutras*, Pajanjali tells us that *Yogah citta vrtti nirodha.* Probably the most often quoted of the aphorisms, this sutra defines yoga as the ability to direct mental activity. Since we live in a culture that believes in a basic distinction between mind and body, spirit and matter, it's difficult at first to see how stretching our spines might affect our thinking. Anyone who engages in regular physical activity, however, understands that exercise brings more blood and oxygen into the tissues, increases neural responsiveness, and releases endorphins to create a sense of well-being. Yoga does all of the above and has the added benefit of releasing negative habit patterns that are stored deep within our tissues.

Etymologically, "yoga" derives from the Sanskrit root *yug,* which means to "yoke, bind, or unite." Hatha yoga combines activity ("ha"/solar energy) with passivity ("tha"/lunar receptivity) to describe a way of working with the physical body that fuses action with restful self-awareness, creating a physiology that is simultaneously strong and flexible. More specifically, Hatha yoga brings the physical body under the intelligent direction of a mind that becomes increasingly sensitive to the body's internal needs. This sensitivity in turn enables a disciplined melding (union) of the mental with the physical that creates and maintains good health. Practicing the physical postures on a regular basis also develops steadiness, lightness of being, clarity of mind, balance, focus and serenity—all signs (according to B. K. S. Iyengar) of "progress on the path of Yoga." Sadhana (practice) creates a positive attitude, bringing both greater physical ease and increased optimism to bear on one's life.

Hatha yoga develops concentration, stillness and—sometimes—the bliss of losing one's self in the process. In this way, it becomes both a comprehensive means of entering a heightened state of awareness and an all-inclusive system of self care. Health and well-being are by-products of the process. They are not the intent. The practice itself is the goal.

* * * * * * * * * * * * * * *

When I was first asked to develop an asana class using the wall for most, if not all, of the poses, I hesitated. Although the Iyengar tradition uses the wall in manifold ways to teach asana, I'm not formally trained in Iyengar teaching methods. I had attended a few restorative classes in which the wall supported students' legs in an effortless *viparita karani*/legs up the wall, and I had been challenged by 2 or 3 hot vinyasa-style classes that focused on hip opening, balance, and the ability to keep one foot on the wall while turning to and away from the center of the room. None of these experiences—taken individually or together—seemed to be enough training for me to adequately develop a series of weekly hour-long classes for students with varying degrees of strength and flexibility.

I pieced the first few sessions together from what I had been taught in Iyengar, restorative and vinyasa classes. As I continued to refine my presentation, I began to ask myself the essential questions every good teacher must answer: "Why am I teaching this material? What do I intend my students to be able to do when they leave class?"

In response to these questions, poses began to reveal themselves. Some appeared as small but necessary steps in preparing the shoulders or hips for some of the complex but foundational poses like warrior I. Some showed themselves to be invaluable aids in developing strength and body awareness. Others built confidence or developed spatial orientation; still others were just fun to do.

About a month after the first class, I had an out-of-town meeting that conflicted with my teaching. A friend and colleague volunteered to sub for me. I told her I'd give her a copy of one of the "flows" (detailed explanations of the poses and their sequences) I often used. While we were talking about the poses, Kathy asked, "Is there a book about this?"

"No," I answered. "I don't think so."

I checked online and in a few bookstores, found nothing and decided to write one. This book is a result of that decision, and, as with many things we set out to do, the journey has been more complex and more interesting than I had at first envisioned. I wrote instructions for about 60 poses and was beginning the introductory material when—"by chance"—I met someone who showed me a few asanas I had missed, opening a door in my thinking that generated new ways to use the wall. Soon I began to see wall poses everywhere. My repertoire grew, but my presentation was choppy. I like classes that flow. Mine did not. Then, as I grew in my own practice, I began to see how poses related one to another—either by general shape or by primary action; as a result of keeping one limb fixed and moving another; or because a joint or muscle group asked to be "countered" by a specific pose in order to restore balance. Little by little, flow happened. . .not for an entire class at first. But discreet sections appeared as I began to see how one pose transformed organically into another. This linking is the foundation on which both my classes and this book are constructed .

As a result of my odyssey, the class that I was reluctant to develop has become a favorite to teach. It's also become a favorite for students for a number of reasons. The wall makes complex poses more available because it's so very there: solid, substantial, unmoving, material. As a result of these properties, the wall tells us where we are in space and gives us feedback about whether or not we're performing the stated actions of a pose—often with surprising results. "I always thought my shoulders were back," one student told me, "until we did triangle at the wall."

We can also use a wall for support until we're strong or balanced enough to work without assistance. Finally, a wall gives us some leverage against the resistance of tight muscles, allowing us to push or pull gently through that resistance in ways we could not do without something concrete to press against.

Through increased appreciation of the body's responses to support, resistance and alignment, we begin to access our personal guru; that is we begin to work with an inner eye to what's "right" and "wrong" for ourselves in each posture—at any given moment. Eventually, we learn to work a pose from the inside out, relying on the teacher within that yoga affirms for each of us.

From classroom to written page is not the easiest journey I've ever made. Nonetheless, my intent has been to create a practical, reader-friendly text that's useful for students and teachers alike. To this end, the material is arranged as follows. The first chapter is largely theoretical.   It's a response to Lynn, a friend and colleague, who suggested I say a little something about what it all means.   Chapter 2 introduces methods of practice and breathing. In the third chapter, you'll find an illustrated discussion of fundamentals: aligning the pelvis, shoulders and spine as well as descriptions of simple movements to encourage joint mobility.

Chapter 4 presents the poses. These are organized into symmetrical and asymmetrical poses based on pelvic position and are further classified by the rotation of the back thigh bone within the hip.   Chapter 4 contains 5 sequences, or flows, that can serve as practice templates.

Not all traditions are in agreement about the importance of the various postures or the order in which they should be practiced. The influences in *Like Stanzas in a Poem: Hatha Yoga at the Wall* come primarily from the teachings of T. Krishnamacharya, through its various streams: Anusara, Ashtanga, Iyengar, Vinyasa and the Yoga of Desikachar.

The title of this book was suggested by Debra Darvick, one of my students, who told me once that, doing yoga at the wall is like stanzas in a poem. Each pose stands by itself but works with the ones that come before and the ones that follow, unfolding the body the way the stanzas of a poem unfold a writer's meaning.

Chapter 1

The Play of Opposites

Without resistance, there is no yoga.

Judith Hanson Lasater

We get by with a little help from our friends.

The Beatles

1

Resistance

Shortly after the publication of *Relax and Renew*, Judith Lasater was touring the country teaching the material in her text. A friend of a friend had studied with her in San Francisco and wanted to reacquaint herself with her former teacher. I had been practicing less than 2 months, it was my first workshop, and Lasater's statement, "Without resistance, there is no yoga," was puzzling. I thought of yoga as a promised bliss of eternal union with the Absolute. I failed to appreciate the complex and often lengthy process whereby we journey from our disharmony into union—first with ourselves, then with other people, and finally, with the life force. In all phases of this journey, resistance plays an important role.

We all know about resistance. We've seen it in ourselves and in others. Within our psyches, it surfaces as an inner "no" that prevents us from looking at painful memories or from facing our fears or from letting go of our past. Or it shows up as dragging our feet when a friend asks for help or a mild belligerence when we suggest that a son or daughter clean their room. We look at most of these experiences as "negative" situations. However, the classical definition given to resistance in physics is a "force that opposes motion" (or current, if you're speaking about electricity). As such, it's neither "good" nor "bad." And in biology, resistance takes on yet another face. Here it's considered healthy since it's defined as an organism's ability to withstand the effects of noxious agents such as bacteria and toxins.

The initial resistance that we face on the yoga mat is physical. Tight muscles and/or rigid joints oppose our movement into a pose. In forward bending, chronically contracted hamstrings resist the flexion of the spine as it folds. When we interlace our fingers behind our back, closed shoulder joints prevent our arms from moving very far away from our sacrum. Working against this kind of resistance through leverage is the primary action of our muscles as they move into and out of yoga postures.

In everyday life, levers are used to lift heavy objects and to pry open stuck lids. Leverage is also the principle whereby muscles stretch and joints develop increased range of motion. By applying force, i.e., muscular effort, at strategic places, we begin to affect the resistances in dense tissues to create movement and change. In the most fundamental of ways, yoga poses are a means of using mechanical advantage (leverage) to open the body.

Muscles work in opposing pairs, so that when one contracts, another stretches. Called agonists and antagonists, they attach to bone near the joints. When a neural impulse stimulates a muscle to shorten, this contraction brings a bone with it, moving a corresponding joint through a particular range of motion in a specific plane. Because improper tracking of the joints results in strain and may lead to injury, the antagonists impede the movement of the agonists, slowing down and smoothing out what might otherwise be a rapid, jerking action. Muscular resistance, therefore, assists stability, keeping joints aligned, so that tendons do not strain or tear, especially if the movement is accompanied by weight bearing. In resisting the movement of the agonists, antagonists protect the joints, the contracting muscle and the tendons that attach muscle to bone. They also promote fluidity and grace.

According to Joel Kramer's article "Yoga as Self-Transformation" in the *Yoga Journal* of May-June 1980, asanas use three different kinds of levers: external (floor, wall); body-on-body (elbow on thigh in spinal twist), and internal (drawing the shoulder blades down the back while reaching up with the hands).

Internal levers, the most difficult to feel and use, require a heightened awareness that develops over time. Working with a wall, a resistant external surface, increases the effectiveness of the body's natural levering by becoming a fixed point against which we press. Working with a wall also helps us become aware of the subtle ways in which micro-movements affect the muscles, connective tissues and joints. In addition to opening the body more effectively, working with a wall fosters awareness of the way internal levers might be used.

The architecture of the body supports the view that yoga is the union of opposites. One muscle contracts concentrically (flexion), drawing itself into the belly of the tissues. Its partner opposes this contraction as in an eccentric stretch (extension). Through attentiveness and repetition, we develop the ability to work this opposition, eventually balancing flexion and extension, drawing in and moving out. Thus resistance is an integral part of change and growth. Tight muscles resist being stretched. Through the work we do with our bodies, muscle tissues break down and repair themselves, adding strength and bulk. Bones are also affected, becoming more dense. As on our mats, so too in our lives—we grow because we look for ways to meet our resistances and to move beyond them.

There's more going on in each pose, however, than mechanical resistance between paired muscle groups. Muscle tissues contract in response to electrical stimuli from the neurons that enervate them. These are largely under the control of our will. However, atrophied or underdeveloped muscles, unforged neural pathways, a lack of kinesthetic awareness, bone structure and injury are all conditions that impede the desired muscular response. This kind of resistance is more subtle than muscular resistance and demands a refined sense of how to

18

work. We modify poses when our range of motion is compromised or when we're not strong enough to do the full asana. We use movement to open joint tissues and to develop kinesthetic awareness. In all cases, using a steady, directed breath, we create a kind of altered state of consciousness, so that we can bring the mind to bear within the tissues of the body.

It's here—in the mind—that we come to see how our resistance to dealing with our *stuff* comes into play in our practice. Our bodies are vast libraries of information. In our DNA, there lives the history of the evolution of our species. In addition, our hips, shoulders, elbows, neck and spine carry the memories that comprise the stories of our individual lives. Each time we experience anything, a biochemical reaction takes place somewhere inside us. If the experience is pleasant, endorphins are released; we feel good. If the experience is not pleasant, we feel sad or angry or frustrated, and corresponding chemicals are released into our blood stream. We feel tired or our stomach gets upset. Our memories are born in this chemical soup, which leaves traces within our cells. Through repetition of particular reactions, we create a palpable psychic residue that becomes part of both our psychological predispositions and our physical structure.

Lower back pain, ulcers, irritable bowel syndrome—many painful chronic conditions are the result of stressful emotions being shunted into our bodies. Working where we're unappreciated, living with a partner who doesn't fully listen, feeling as though we need to do better and be better than we are in order to be loved—all of these are fairly common situations. And all of them deliver a more or less steady stream of toxic chemicals into our tissues. Although we are all too aware—if we take the time to look—of our life situations and our feelings about them, most of us are not aware of the bio-chemical reactions that take place below the radar of our conscious mind. They surface only when their effects have become so deeply ingrained that we've created dis-ease.

One of the basic principles on which we human creatures operate is the pursuit of pleasure and the avoidance of pain. Shunting emotions into the body is one mechanism by which many of us avoid the discomfort of difficult, negative feelings. This fundamental psychic resistance is the fodder for any meaningful yoga practice as we work with our bodies to unlock the mysteries of our minds and our emotions. We may find, for example, that working with pigeon pose not only opens the psoas, but it also uncovers a deep sorrow over the loss of a lover. Or we may find that the chronic discomfort around our right shoulder stems from feeling as though we're bearing the weight of the world. Most of us would rather avoid poses that open us up to the psychic pain we've spent so much time avoiding, and psychic resistance often proves to be more intransigent than tight hamstrings. Over time, however, we come to appreciate the effectiveness of yoga in dealing with our "stuff" and to develop a fascination with what will come up next. Through asana we see that our mind does not exist in isolation from our body; rather, these two—body and mind—are inextricably connected. Yoga is more than a tool for stretching our hamstrings; it's a technology for understanding our minds and hearts.

While pain and dis-ease are often caused by our unwillingness to deal with heartache and disappointment, it's also true that there are times when a stomach ache can show us areas of our lives in which greater resistance needs to be cultivated. When presented with a situation that's potentially harmful—as in the field of biology so too in human life—resistance becomes a paradigm for health. Our yoga practice helps us here too. Through it we develop the ability to discern the difference between resistance that impedes and that which assists our growth.

When we take a long, hard look at the pain we've locked up inside ourselves—whether it be in our joints or stomach or mind, we begin to see patterns. For instance, perhaps we never got on well with our mother. Was she inherently unsympathetic or too harried to give us the attention we wanted? Either way, as we grew, we got used to the way she treated us; we built a wall around ourselves to protect us from the pain of wanting more intimacy than we got. We fell in love, married and discovered—to our dismay—that the person we married was just like our mom—unable to fully appreciate us or too busy to care. When the secrets we keep hidden from ourselves surface on the yoga mat, we see that our past conditions determine our present circumstances

This is a "no-brainer" for anyone involved in a 12-step program or for many of us who've participated in counseling. What IS miraculous is that we can choose not to participate in the patterns we've grown accustomed to. As we address our issues, we release their hold. Our habits change. Instead of picking a fight or finding solace in a piece of chocolate or a cup of coffee when we're feeling unloved, we find something positive to do for ourselves. We paint or hop on our bicycle or get onto the yoga mat. Healthy habits don't grow overnight. Neither does a positive attitude. Instead, they strobe. Sometimes we're bright and strong. At other times we're feeling quite strong but are without a light. At still others, we have neither strength nor light; the pattern has reasserted itself. Then, when we feel that it's all been a wash, we find our path again.

Coming into yoga is a process. Eventually we reach a clearing in the woods next to the bank of a stream. A boat meanders downstream towards us, carrying an opportunity to repeat the pattern we've been working so hard to eliminate. We look inside ourselves to find there is not one trace of longing to board the boat. We know where it will go, and it was never good. We have developed immunity, the kind of resistance defined by biology as the ability to withstand that which will hurt us.

20

Mechanical, mental-emotional, biological—these 3 forms of resistance are inherent to our yoga—a liberating practice that unites us with something beyond ourselves. As we work with the resistance in our physical bodies, we stretch and strengthen and we also open ourselves to greater understanding. Unearthing what we would rather resist in ourselves can be a life's work. But from it we can learn many things about our patterns, about our lives and about what we might be. As we practice, we become immune to the pull of situations that keep us stuck, and we become more open to those experiences that increase peace, joy and wisdom. In other words, we work with and learn from the resistances within us. Without them, there is no process and there is no yoga.

Support

At the same time I was introduced to yoga, I was also reading the first three books by Carlos Castaneda that describe shamanic practices indigenous to native people of northern Mexico. One of the central concepts was the existence of the antiphonal pair of spirits known as the adversary and the ally. An adversary is one who, by virtue of his or her antagonism, makes us stronger. An ally, as we all know, is someone who is on our side.

Resistance and support work in much the same fashion—both on and off the mat. We need a little help from things that are challenging—other people, our inner demons, stiff backs—to keep us awake; we need to be able to rely on external forces—on other people and on props—to support us when we're too tired or too weak or too "whatever" to make it on our own. Consider the following.

At the periphery of the practice room, 10 students are seated on the floor. Their ankles or shins are crossed. Their knees tilt at 45° angles toward the ceiling. Their spines, rounded at the shoulder blades, rest on the wall behind them. Two to three times a week these same people, most of them over 65, meet at the studio to stretch, strengthen and work on balance. In the aerobics room at a local health club, 13 women in various stages of pregnancy stand with their right hands lightly touching the wall. Bellies ballooning forward, left feet touching their right thighs or calves, they balance in tree pose. Across town at another studio, half a dozen people are turned upside down. Their hands hug the floor; their backs face the wall, and their feet, elevated above their heads, lightly touch the wall behind them. For all of these people, the wall is a welcome means of support.

Support is the most obvious of the several ways a wall can be useful in an asana class. It helps us maintain balance until our muscles are strong and our nervous systems developed enough so that we no longer wobble or fall when we move away. On the mat, as in life, balance can be a difficult dance. On the one hand, we don't want to rely too much on a prop; we might become habituated to its use and never develop the strength or neural connections to work on our own. On the other, we don't want to let go before we're ready. A fall might lead to injury. *Then* where would we be?

We live in a culture that encourages us to be disconnected from our feet and from our lower bodies. We sit in cars and on furniture that's too soft to keep us awake and aware. We work at desks where we round forward toward a computer screen. We wear shoes that deprive our toes of the space they need to work independently. And we shut away pelvic and inner thigh sensations because of their association with a sexuality of which we're taught to be suspicious. Compounding matters, we live in our heads, thinking incessantly about where we've been and what might happen tomorrow. We play video games, watch television, chat on the internet. All of these activities contribute to legs and hips that are only partially awake. Our weight distributes unevenly, putting undue pressure on one hip or the other. Toes curl in or a knee turns out, and joints begin to wear down under repeated stress.

Standing is a commonplace but complex process. We take it for granted but most of us don't do it well. We're unaware of how our weight is distributed on our feet or through our joints. The left foot presses harder into the earth than the right. Or we settle a little more into the right or the left hip. Seldom do we think about how we hold ourselves upright until we begin to experience problems. Painful toes, stiff knees and sore hips draw our attention to our weight bearing habits.

The very same tendencies that contribute to an unconscious lower body make standing balance poses hard for many of us to do. When told to raise our right foot even a few inches off the earth, we wobble from side to side. We find it nearly impossible to stand for even one breath with the ball of the left foot fully connected to the ground. As we age, a life time of bad habits increases our precariousness. A wall is a good friend at such times. For people with more serious conditions— multiple sclerosis, vertigo, partial tissue atrophy—a wall is invaluable. In pregnancy, where balance is thrown off because of increased weight gain in the front plane of the body, a wall can also be a source of stability.

Once the body is stable, learning can begin. The foot learns how to maintain contact with the floor. The quads learn to lift and hold the knee in place. The adductors learn to work with the psoas to keep the pelvis supple but firm. The postural muscles learn to hold the vertebrae in line. The use of support is thus a fundamental step in an educational process that leads us toward achieving autonomy. On the mat, as in life, the process of coming into balance begins with perceiving how and what we're doing and then using what's available to help us strengthen those areas of ourselves that need to be developed. Once they've been retrained to

22

be more vital, they function without support to sustain integrity and wholeness.

From the simplest toe raise to the more complex half moon to the arduous handstand, the wall can create a window of freedom from the fear of falling. Without fear and the tremor associated with trying to keep ourselves erect, we're more easily able to concentrate on learning to balance. The scenarios that follow exemplify ways to use the wall for support in a variety of typical class situations.

Scenario 1. An attractive brunette in her early 50s comes to class once a week. Her legs are flaccid and seem to be disconnected from the rest of her. Due to multiple sclerosis, this once-active woman can barely climb the steps to the studio. In the same class, a jaunty 75-year-old man, muscles toned from years of tennis, wobbles on feet crippled by bunions. Standing next to him is a 32-year-old woman with a closed head injury that makes her dizzy and gives her intermittent headaches. For all of these people, a simple leg raise can be both helpful and perilous. For each of these people, a wall is an invaluable friend.

"Progress" can be hard to detect. Depending on the severity of a student's condition, it might take her months or even years before she's able to stand on one foot without the support of the wall. The ability to do so is not necessarily the point. Breathing within the framework of where we are, creating balance with or without assistance, being more present and alive—these are the goals as well as the benefits.

Scenario 2. The class is smaller than usual, but the students who've come are not inexperienced. They've been practicing for several years and are able to stand steadily on one foot for an extended period of time. They're strong, familiar with triangle and warrior 2, and have moderately open shoulders and hips. They like challenges; it's time to learn to fly. Half moon pose, ardha chandrasana, is the perfect vehicle for this.

Ardha chandrasana with the back at the wall is the best example I know of the way in which support leads to growth and freedom. The ability to lean back and lift up out of the pelvis and standing leg develops trust and an other-worldly sense of being freed from the gravitational pull of the earth. We become, if only for a few breaths, lighter and more buoyant.

Scenario 3: As a group, the students in the 6:15 Tuesday and Thursday evening class approach their practice with a sense of adventure. Often coming to the studio directly from work they release that tired, day's-end feeling into the earth through their postures. Their down dogs are strong; their shoulders are open; they're eager to try new things. Handstand against the wall gives them a new perspective. One of my childhood friends told me she thought everyone should spend some time each day upside down. It changes the way we view the world and brings some playfulness into our lives. It also builds confidence and upper body strength. It energizes body and spirit.

Scenario 4: Tired from a long week at work, Carol, a marketing manager, places the short edge of her mat next to the wall. She lies down and brings her legs above her so that her ankles, knees, and hips stack one above the other. Her hands rest on her abdomen. Her eyes close. She sinks into herself, allowing gravity to draw the fatigue from her feet and legs. This pose, a variation of *viparita karani,* reverse action, is a classic restorative pose that uses the wall for support so that the body can rest. Here there is no need for balance or for work There's no need for learning for that matter. The purpose of the pose is to return vitality to the tissues and to rejuvenate the spirit.

For a long time, I was an "I-can-handle-it" kind of girl. Driven by a need to prove myself as well as by a reluctance to be beholden to anyone, I refused most offers of help. I often worked longer than I had to on projects because I didn't want to inconvenience anyone by asking for or accepting a helping hand. When I first began practicing yoga, I carried this spirit of independence into my practice. I was a "no prop" snob. Blocks, straps, blankets and bolsters were too cumbersome to carry with me, and they impeded the flow of my practice. They were things for other, less-able students, to use. I saw props as crutches along the path toward personal growth, not aids along the way.

Within the past few years, however, I've come to understand that receiving help does not belittle or confine me. One needs to be open in order to prosper, and being willing to receive the loving support of others is an important component of this openness. Throughout our lives, support comes in many forms. Sometimes we need a loan of money or furniture or perhaps a car when ours is in for repairs. Often, however, we just need someone who has enough faith in our vision to help us bring it out from the ethereal realms of wishful thinking and into the reality of daily life. Whatever form support takes for us, a willingness to recognize that we need help is prerequisite.

For everything there is a season. When we first begin to learn to balance on one foot or on our hands, we need a little help—from a wall or a trusted teacher. As we grow stronger and more able, we learn to balance, to ride the currents of our lives without holding on. It's then that we can safely let go. . .of the wall, of the hand that was offered, of the prop that served as a stepping stone, of the internal resistance to change that we thought would keep us safe. Antagonists and agonists, adversaries and allies, resistance and support--all reflect the theme. The union of opposites--this is yoga.

Chapter 2

Opening and Inspiration —

How to Practice and Breathe

The aim of the yoga is to contact the Inner Psychic and from there to act increasingly on the outer world.

Sri Aurobindo

The real voyage of discovery consists not of seeking new landscapes but of having new eyes.

Marcel Proust

2

Being Open

Openness.

We hear a lot about it. We're told to be "open" to the universal good, to be "open" to others, to be "open" to our inner self worth. Yet what, exactly, does it mean to be open? More importantly, how do we do it?

On the yoga mat, being open generally means that our joints are spacious enough to accommodate a particular range of motion. Or it might mean that we're receptive to a particular set of instructions and/or suggestions. Our minds grasp, our muscles "take," and our nervous systems integrate the directions. Moving yoga off the mat, "being open" might mean that we listen attentively to what our roommate or spouse or children have to say about us, especially if it comes in the form of criticism. It could also mean that we might try a Thai restaurant when we haven't ever eaten in one before or that we follow the advice of a respected confidant about how to conduct our personal, business or financial affairs.

These openings, however important, are all aspects of a more profound process. According to the most prevalent metaphor, yoga "opens" those who practice much as one peels away the skins of an onion to uncover an ever more pungent substance inside. Thus, for the yogi, openness is about delving beneath the surface of our everyday lives and the roles and responsibilities these lives bring. For the yogi, being open is a continual process of shedding limits, of letting go. We let go of our identification with our roles, for example. Being a parent or a teacher or an engineer or a student—all require commitments of time and energy. But defining ourselves by our ability to take care of others or solve complex problems closes us to a more interesting reality. And so does our identification with the adjectives that attached themselves to us as children and followed us into adulthood. We may be cute or stubborn or easy to get along with, but we are more than that. Our true identity is far more complex than our attributes or the roles we fulfill in daily life. The key to experiencing this lies deep inside, in the Self.

Some say this Self, the *jivatman*, sits in our hearts in the form of a soul, no bigger than a thumb. Some say that the Self is no thing at all; rather it is a current of consciousness that, co-extensive with the universal energetic intelligence, runs throughout our entire form.

Regardless of the way this Self is described, yoga tells us that the ego is but its house. Our roles in the world and our accomplishments—so much a part of our ego identification and our sense of personal worth—are little more than clothing for the inner spark that is simultaneously distinguished from and at union with the force that infuses all of creation.

Yoga, then, is a technique that undresses us so that we can find our inner light.

Sometimes, however, the undressing feels more like a dressing down. We come to class to find that the marathon training we've undertaken has tightened our hamstrings so much that we're unable to do even the simplest forward bend, let alone any of the more complex poses that "everyone" around us is doing. Or, while stepping forward into a lunge, we experience an opening in our psoas that triggers a memory of a traumatic breakup with a former lover. Or we find that the music our teacher plays at the end of class brings up a loneliness we thought we'd left behind. Here it is again, and we're overwhelmed. At such times, being open is not the promised bliss. But it *is* part of the process.

Socialization requires us to defer difficult emotions such as sorrow, jealousy, anger and frustration so that we can amicably live with those around us. By the time we're young adults, we become conditioned to shoving down unpleasant feelings. Some of us are so good at deflecting negative emotions that we no longer feel them. Our bodies, however, do. Muscles become tight, joints lose range of motion, jaws set, faces grow pinched. This kind of armoring becomes our "natural" state.

In removing tension from muscle tissues through asana practice, yoga not only opens us to stored memories, it also teaches us about our programming. We begin to see, for example, that we never assert ourselves, choosing instead some passive form of directing aggression toward those with whom we disagree. We "accidentally" drop an expensive new camera or show up late for a meeting. Or we see that whenever someone offers us a suggestion our shoulders hunch, our jaw tightens and we listen with half an ear instead of our full attention, blocking what could be helpful because we're too stubborn to admit that we need assistance. Once we begin to observe our "stuff," we can also begin to let it go. This leads to increased internal space—a space in which we begin to experience the kind of freedom from programming that begets both generosity and compassion.

Our habitual reactions keep us in a kind of prison, looking at the external world through the various filters of our likes and dislikes. These filters press against the people and circumstances that surround us, distorting them. As we progress in our yoga, we begin to experience a deactivation of our habits. When someone cuts us off in traffic, for example, we realize we don't have to shout or lay on the horn or raise our hand in reply. We can let the energy of the car and driver move past us without getting caught in it. We might even wish the driver a bit of goodwill.

Of course, most of us will not, in one class or even in one lifetime, peel away all the layers we've wrapped around ourselves in this and previous incarnations. Nor should we think that completely disrobing, standing naked before the wind, is or should be the goal of our practice. We need a bit of ego to live our lives.

Sometimes, however, in the spaciousness that we create, we're able to feel the breath of the universal consciousness. *Paramatman* (highest, supreme soul) is its name; Emerson called it the Oversoul. Many traditions call it love—the intelligence that suffuses and nurtures all things. Whatever it is, it's there for us. It seeps into the spaciousness our practice provides. It informs our vision; we begin to see people and circumstances as reflections of a benevolent face. Even that which is difficult becomes an occasion for growth.

This is the openness that yoga cultivates. It is, as Sri Aurobindo, the founder of Integral Yoga, tells us, the "inner psychic" acting ever more on the outside world. The more we peel away the layers, the more we can connect with the consciousness that infuses creation. The more we connect with this light of Spirit, the lighter we feel and the more brightly we can shine for ourselves and others.

To this end—connecting more brightly to the inner light—observe the following guidelines for your physical practice:

How to Practice

Where: Practice in a clean, well lit room. Natural light is best since it's not as hard on the eyes as incandescent or fluorescent lighting. The ambient temperature should be at least 70 degrees. Heat brings blood into muscle tissues, helping prevent injury. Some yoga traditions require 80 and 90 degree rooms for practice. If you're used to such heat, by all means, crank it up. If not, make sure the air is warm enough so that you don't feel cold while you're at rest in your shirt sleeves. Wear any comfortable clothing that allows movement and makes you feel good about yourself.

When: Most yoga books suggest a daily practice at the same hour each day. This conditions the body, keeping it healthy much as taking a daily vitamin after breakfast assures that you will get the required nutrients to remain energetic all day long. A morning practice dissipates any tension brought about by dreams or mental processing during sleep. It also gets the blood circulating and opens the joints for greater comfort throughout the day. One teacher says, "An hour after rising, do your yoga." Given the hectic nature of our lives, this is not entirely

28

practicable advice, and evening practice can dissolve the day's worries and create an inner calm before bed.

Regardless of the time of day, allow at least 3 hours to elapse after eating a heavy meal before you begin to perform the asanas. This lets your stomach clear (making forward bending much more comfortable and releasing blood for your muscles). Because asana practice competes for your energy, do not practice when you have a fever. A mild head cold may feel better through practice, however. Most teachers caution menstruating and pregnant women not to do inversions.

How Often and How Long: Whatever your schedule allows. Do the best you can. In the beginning work with the poses 2 to 3 times per week whenever you have the time. Monitor your energy and activity levels and adjust your practice accordingly. Although the "usual" Yoga studio class lasts from 60-90 minutes, feel free to do less or more as your time and energy allow. Even 15-20 minutes a couple of times a week will give a marked improvement in your sense of well-being. For real progress toward becoming open, however, a daily practice is best.

What (to Practice):

1. Practice a single pose, one of the flows included in Chapter 5, or a sequence of your own design. Individual poses can be used to supplement a more traditional, non-wall practice, cultivating skills and opening tissues for hard-to-access asanas. We all have them, and they're different for each of us.

2. Work with the instructions as guidelines rather than as fixed rules. Above all work with your breath and with your own internal guidance to find your way through the complexity within this book and others like it. The number of breaths recommended in each sequence is conventional but also somewhat arbitrary. Conventions vary: an even number of breaths come from Viniyoga and the Yoga of Desikachar; odd numbers of breaths come from ashtanga. Neither is sacred; rather they seem to align with feminine (even) and masculine (odd) orientations.

3. Cultivate sensitivity to the differences between mental and physical resistance. Honor each (it serves to protect you from potential harm—imagined or real). But don't give in to either. Rather explore the resistance. Breathe into it until it begins to dissolve. This may take only a few minutes; sometimes, however, it takes days or years. Be patient and loving toward yourself.

4. Be creative. The number of breaths and the number of repetitions for each asana are suggestive, not prescriptive. Allow yourself the freedom to pick and choose the poses and methods that fit your needs. Use the basic ingredients of breath and leverage, check in to discover what you need to be doing for your body or your students at any given time, set a destination and discover new ways to get there. Yoga is above all experiential. The body is your laboratory, so approach your practice with a sense of adventure.

5. Muscles learn in at least two primary ways. Repetition establishes neuro-muscular patterning. Holding a pose triggers muscular corrections at the site of localized pressure, i.e., where leverage is applied. Decide what your goal is in each asana, or for a particular practice, and adjust the poses accordingly: hold longer or shorter; do more repetitions or fewer.

6. To understand your own breathing patterns and to begin to coordinate this breathing into a useful measure for yourself, see how many cycles of inhalation and exhalation you take in a minute. Slow your breath down and recount. Play with faster and slower counts to experience the effects of each and adjust your rhythms according to desired outcomes for a particular pose or session.

7. Work with either a fixed gaze (a *drishti*) or with your eyes closed. A fixed gaze alters your visual field, which in turn diverts mental activity from its normal patterns. This makes way for a more meditative, mindful performance of the pose. A *drishti* additionally helps us with our alignment since the head must be held at a particular angle in order to maintain the gaze at a particular point.

   Working with the eyes closed, however, encourages a person to tune into sensation. This helps some people learn more about the effects of each pose *from the inside out*, increasing conscious proprioception and encouraging an understanding of how and why to make slight adjustments so that the pose is at once more engaging and more comfortable.Unfortunately neither using a gaze point nor closing the eyes works all the time for all people, so experiment. The important thing to remember is to focus on what you're doing on your mat instead of what you did before you began to practice or what you'll do when you're finished.

Overall, allow yourself to be inspired. Working with the miracle of your body in asana is a journey into an amazing landscape of sinew, bone, muscle and memory. Don't fret about trying to be "better" at poses. Instead, forget about your destination and enjoy the ride.

Inspiration

If you can't use either a gaze point or closed eyes to let go of household chores, yesterday's golf game or your sagging thighs, put on some music and allow your mind to entrain to the rhythm or the beat. Or, if that doesn't silence your inner dialogue, explore some of the options that follow. Each tradition has its own ways of engaging the mind in asana. Some use visualization; some employ sound (mantra); still others combine energies, using both.

Specific visualizations vary with traditions, but they can be divided into two primary types--for ourselves and for others. When we imagine ourselves doing a handstand or stretching into the splits, we're visualizing. Given the broad scope of yoga, this might seem like a superficial and/or egotistically self-serving procedure. Nonetheless, suppleness, lightness of being, and balance are all conditions of the yogic experience. As such they're legitimate subjective experiences and, for those of us who have a fear of being upside down or are convinced only the "other" gender has the proper ligamentation to open the groins in splits, visualizing ourselves in "impossible' postures is huge. It's the first step toward moving beyond limitation. In this way, seeing ourselves in poses we can't currently perform leads us also to overcome mental limitations.

There are numerous other ways to use visualizations in asana practice to overcome limitations—to encourage us to be more open. Chief among them are using a theme; i.e., focusing on being truthful with ourselves as we move in and out of poses, or practicing non-violence by easing into and out of poses instead of forcing our bodies beyond their edge. These qualities, when we use them consciously throughout a session, train us to think more compassionately and honestly in our everyday lives.

Working with images of energy is another way that visualizations assists us on the mat. We can, for instance, imagine a golden ball of light moving up and down our spines as we breathe. Or, when we raise our arms above our head, we can "see" clear lines of energy moving from the earth's core through our feet, up our legs and torso and out the crown of our head and our fingertips to merge with the universal life force. Thus we visualize ourselves merging with both earth and sky, and we become more open on an energetic level.

A second type of visualization is done for the benefit of others. Here we use our powers of imaging to manifest good in the lives of people who are suffering or otherwise in need of compassion. At the beginning of practice, we dedicate our efforts to another by bringing them clearly to mind, placing them on the mat with or in front of us, and consistently thinking about them as we bend and twist and lunge. Because many of us will work harder for someone else than for ourselves, this method has a two-fold benefit. First, our minds are powerful tools, and dedicating our practice to another "sends" that person some good energy, which has the potential to help them physically and spiritually. Secondly, through the practice itself, we become more flexible, more charitable and more in tune with ourselves as members of a community.

Although visualization is a stellar way to bring us inspiration on the mat, not everyone finds it easy to call up images. Some of us respond much more readily to sound. If this is your situation, you might find that using mantras will take you more deeply into inner space.

Loosely speaking, whenever we repeat anything over and over to ourselves, we're saying a mantra. Thus, to the extent that visualization uses words to carry the images we employ, mantra is also the vehicle for our visualizations. If we say, for example, "I am happy. I'm relaxed. I am happy. I'm relaxed. I am happy. I'm relaxed" throughout our practice, inhaling and exhaling with each sentence, we become happy and relaxed. This occurs whether or not we actually "see" ourselves smiling and at ease because our subconscious can (and does) do the imaging for us.

In the 1960s and 'early 1970s, when the Beatles became initiated into Transcendental Meditation, "mantra" was defined as "meaningless sound." A look at the word's origins, however, suggests another definition. Etymologically, *mantra* is derived from the Sanskrit root *man-*, "to think" and *–tra*, which denotes a tool or a process. So a mantra is a mind tool or the act/process of thinking. A friend of mine has called it a "mind protector," since repeating a mantra more or less effectively prevents us from thinking other things; in particular, it can keep us off the hamster wheel of obsessively negative thought patterns.

"Mantra" originally referred to entire portions of Hindu scriptures that were rendered in poetic form. In both esoteric and mundane Hindu practices, mantra became the form that desire and will took *en route* to manifestation. Because of its vibratory properties, the universe and all things within it are said to have evolved from sound. Thus, the Sanskrit syllables that comprise a mantra are considered to carry the power of manifestation, that is they are able to bring things into being. This power can be spiritual as in *Lokah samastah sukhino bhavnathu*: May all the beings in all the worlds become happy. Or it can have the properties of an incantation, encouraging personal prosperity and happiness. On a psychological level, repeating mantras develops one-pointedness, the ability to concentrate—which, in our fast-paced culture full of distractions--is one of the true gifts of yoga.

Mantra and visualization can both be used to quiet a racing mind. Another tool is with us all the time. It's our breath.

Although we all breathe, most of us don't do it well. In stressful situations we either hold our breaths or we hyperventilate—often without any awareness that we're doing so. Whether stuck in traffic when we're late for work, making a point in conversation with someone who has a different opinion, or learning how to operate a new computer program, if we pay attention to our breathing, we'll probably find that it has been changed by the stress of what we're trying to accomplish.

One of the first bits of yoga lore I learned was that each of us is given a specific number of breaths during our lives. The more slowly we breathe, therefore, the longer we'll live. Whether this is true or not, in asana practice, the more slowly we breathe, the more closely we can pay attention to what's happening in our bodies. This in turn enables us to work attentively and to open our tissues in an organic, mindful way. Paying attention to our respiration, taking slow, deliberate, even breaths can—in and of itself—without mantra or visualization—calm the chatter of our minds and bring us into a more one-pointed, meditative awareness. It encourages what's known as "witness consciousness," a state of mind from which we can both watch and participate in what we experience.

Of all of the practices in Hatha Yoga, the cultivation of a measured breath is perhaps the most important. Yoga differs from other forms of physical activity in that the mind is an essential component. One does not read the newspaper or watch television while practicing— and with good reason. Awareness is essential to get the most out of each asana and to avoid injury. The breath, so vital for life, is also vital for practice in that it helps us to participate fully in what we're doing.

During my own practice, I nearly always use some form of Ujjayi breathing (see p. 38), but the yogic or the diaphragmatic breaths (see p. 37) are also fine if either feels more comfortable to you. The only stipulation is that you work in the following manner: if you can feel your heart or pulse beating, use its rhythm to count—4, 6 or 8 (or longer) for each inhalation and the same for each exhalation. If you're not able to feel the rhythm of your heart, then tap lightly with your mind in equal intervals to make the count. The more steadily we breathe within and between poses, the more deeply we can experience the internal work that transpires. A 6-8 count rhythm is sufficiently slow (based on a pulse of 60 beats per minute) to create a meditative state, yet it is also energizing enough to support an asana practice.

How to Breathe

3-Part Yogic Breath

This type of breathing is taught in many beginning yoga classes. It frees the diaphragm and encourages a deeper inspiration than is normal for most of us. It can be done seated on the floor, in a chair or lying face up on a hard surface. Until it becomes your natural state of breathing, do it lying down.

Before you begin, take a moment to observe the mechanics of your normal breath. Notice what portion of your front body moves on your inhale—belly, upper chest wall, shoulders. Notice, too, whether the movement expands this area or contracts it. As babies we naturally breath into our bellies, expanding this area with the in-breath and allowing it to sink in (contract) on the out-breath. Because we live in a belly-phobic culture, many of us, by the time we reach our teens, are breathing paradoxically, that is we contract our abdomens on the inhale. This results in frustration for the diaphragm, diminishing the space inside the chest cavity for the lower lobes of the lungs. If this is the breathing pattern that seems most natural to you, the following methods may be difficult at first. Be patient. Change doesn't take place overnight. There may come a moment when the confusion between what you intend and what you're doing becomes intense. Be calm, visualize the new way, and allow your body to move toward it.

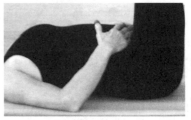

1. Begin by lying on the floor with your feet on the wall and your knees over your hips. Place your hands on your abdomen, just below your navel.

2. As you inhale, consciously press your abdomen into your hands. Feel your diaphragm expand into the region of your internal organs. Feel the curvature of your lower back expand as well. It may flatten lightly against the floor. Exhale by releasing your diaphragm; allow your stomach and hands to sink toward your spine. Repeat as many as 10 times.

3. Next, move both hands to your ribs and as you inhale, consciously breathe into your palms, feeling lift with the expansion of your diaphragm. Here you've moved your inspiration into the mid-regions of your lungs. Feel your ribs—front and back—expand as well. Repeat as many as 10 times.

4. Move both your hands to your upper chest wall and breathe into the upper regions of your lungs, seeing if you can feel movement in your hands. Keep your breath high and shallow for up to 10 breaths.

5. Put it all together as you inhale and exhale, filling each region successively. Breathing in this fashion does more than create optimal space for the expansion of your lungs. Your diaphragm is attached to your ribs, sternum and spine. At rest it sits directly above your stomach, spleen, kidneys, liver, and pancreas. Complete breathing not only massages your spine, helping to maintain spinal mobility, and it also gently massages your internal organs.

Diaphragmatic Breath

This breath draws attention to the middle of the body, to the core. It's useful for asana practice because it fosters awareness of the thoracic cavity and the chest wall and because it creates an effective support for the lumbar spine. Work with it once you've become familiar with the 3-part yogic breath. Begin in a comfortable, supine position, but with both hands on your ribs.

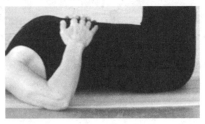

1. Exhale completely but without strain. Feel your abdomen draw in toward your spine and your diaphragm lift toward your heart and lungs.

2. Maintaining a slight contraction in your lower belly (known as uddiyana bandha in the ashtanga tradition), draw your diaphragm into this resistance.

3. Feel your ribs expand—to the sides, front, back—and telescope, one from the other, toward your chin. Keep your shoulders relaxed while your chest expands.

4. To exhale, draw your diaphragm and upper abdominal muscles in and up. You may feel a slight movement in your shoulders as well as in your neck and head. And you may notice your attention move more deeply inward.

5. Repeat steps 4 and 5, paying attention to the resistance in your lower abdomen, which refers the diaphragmatic expansion into your ribs and upper chest wall.

Ujjayi Pranayama Breath

This is also known as Conquering, So-Hum and Ocean Breath. Technically it's a form of Pranayama (breath regulation) but--unlike other forms of breathing exercises--can be safely practiced any time and anywhere throughout the day.

1. Begin with diaphragmatic breathing. On your exhalation, open your mouth and say "haaaaa." Notice the sensation at the back of your throat. Repeat.

2. After your next inhalation, say "haaaaa" again, but with your mouth closed. Your exhalation will be generated from your glottis.

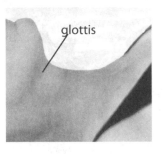

glottis

3. Draw your next inhalation into your lungs in the same fashion—into the back of your throat. The sound of the constricted air flow on the inhalation is similar to a deep and prolonged "aaaaaaah."

4. Do ujjayi breathing for 10 breaths or up to 5 minutes, and observe the sensations in your body and the effects the breathing has on your mental processes.

Inspiration is an essential component of respiration, the process whereby our cells are oxygenated and waste products such as carbon dioxide and water are carried away. It's also a part of learning to be more open. Finding peace, getting off of our mental hamster wheels— both of these are necessary in order to discover a sweeter Self inside the layers of our life roles and our egos. Without letting go, there is no room for inspiration or for breath. Without inspiration, without breath—neither cells nor psyche can live.

Chapter 3

When Less Is More: Fundamentals

So much depends/ upon /a red wheel/ barrow/ glazed with rain/ water/ beside the white/ chickens.

William Carlos Williams

3

Yoga's emphasis on the spine is one of its hallmarks. Without a healthy, flexible spinal column, nerves become pinched, mobility is impaired and pain becomes a constant companion. Nothing, however, exists in isolation. This is as true within the structures of our bodies as it is in the natural world. And so, a healthy spine requires healthy hips and shoulders as well as fully functioning limbs. Yoga, therefore, works with the entire body to cultivate supple muscles and freely moving joints. To this end, symmetry and balance are important principles to take into consideration as we move and position our bodies, as is our relationship to the earth and its gravitational field. Gravity is heavy (pun intended). It keeps us attached to the earth, this is true, but it's also a force against which we act on a daily basis.

Mechanically, the body is a wonder. Tiny vertebrae stack, one atop another, to form the human spine. Muscles layer and interweave, change form and merge with chord-like tendons and, eventually, with ligaments that attach to bones in a series of levers and pulleys that, defying the downward pull of gravity, enables us to bear weight and to move. Arms, trunk and legs are strategically segmented and hinged so that we can bend and twist and turn. Called the *rectus abdominis* at the front and *erector spinae* behind, the muscles of the trunk keep us upright. At each end of the spine, the pelvic and shoulder girdles transfer weight and movement from the trunk to the limbs and from the limbs to the trunk.

Our feet interface between our physical selves and the earth upon which they tread. Structurally, our arches are designed to distribute body weight evenly across our feet, but genetic predispositions and the wear and tear of life dispose the design toward malfunction. Flat feet, bunions, heel spurs—these are painful reminders that our feet are important to our well being. Foot problems generally indicate that there's also something amiss with one or more of our knees and hips; the spine and shoulders may also suffer pain and/or misalignment when our feet are not happily carrying us on our daily rounds.

Because of the lifestyle common in developed nations—spending untold hours seated on chairs and sofas—our pelvic and shoulder girdles are often as miserable as our feet. The downward pull of gravity takes its toll as hips bear the constant pressure of our sedentary lives. Our shoulders, while not so much affected by gravity, are nonetheless victims of our everyday activities. While we sit at the keyboard or at the wheel of the car, our arms move forward, taking our shoulders with them. As a result, our spines begin to lose their natural curves to take on other, less healthy shapes, and we begin to hurt.

Pain is one of our most time-honored teachers. Many of us won't consider making changes in our diets or lifestyles unless and until we begin to hurt somewhere. This is as true for many of us who come to yoga as it for those who seek medical treatment. The first step to alleviating pain is understanding its cause. To this end, this chapter presents detailed information and exercises to bring us in touch with fundamental principles of aligning the pelvis, shoulders, feet and hands. It also presents some guidelines for generating good posture—optimum spinal alignment—while sitting and standing.

The exercises are simple. But don't be fooled by this. Each fosters a critical awareness that's foundational to daily life as well as to the poses that follow and to the poses in the general body of asanas being practiced in most hatha yoga classes today. The exercises in this chapter are well suited for those of advanced years, and they're excellent for working with injuries. Each can also be used to introduce a central concept/skill toward the beginning of a class for people of varying age and mobility.

Jonny Kest, my first teacher, is fond of saying that the only difference between you and the person who's taking a deeper twist or a more advanced version of a pose is that they need to go a little farther to find their edge. If we're practicing mindfully, the edge can be elusive and ever changing. Some days we don't find it in a seated forward bend until our head rests on our shins. On other days we barely begin to move our torsos forward and we find it—it's that place that says "Oops. Don't go any further or you'll be sorry." For each of us it's a slightly different place and for many of us it's a slightly different place on different days.

Nonetheless, the edge is the place where we want to work. Pay close attention to where you feel the effects of the pose and where you don't. Begin to learn when you're working too hard and when you're not doing enough. Even in the most basic of postures, there's an optimal mixture of comfort, awareness and muscular effort. Learn to use your breath to determine where this is in each and every pose. Take a few minutes to establish an even breath, and practice in such a way that you maintain continuity in its rhythm.

Synthesizing the wealth of teaching about technique for each pose is no easy task. In general, however, we work with the following caveats:

1. Knees and elbows should not be torqued. Because of this, especially in weight-bearing poses, ankles, knees and hips should "track" in the same plane. This is also true of wrists, elbows and shoulders.

2. Bones bear weight most efficiently when they're perpendicular to the ground. This is another reason to align our joints.

3. Keeping our lower abdominal muscles slightly contracted (drawn in toward our spine) supports the lower back.

4. Drawing the shoulder blades towards each other and down the back expands the chest wall, increasing space for our lungs. It also protects the fragile shoulder joints in weight-bearing circumstances.

5. Telescoping ribs up away from our hips (keeping the "side bodies long") also expands our breathing room. In addition, it redistributes the force of our body's weight on the pelvis.

6. Engaging the inner thigh muscles decompresses the sacrum while contributing to pelvic stability.

7. In standing poses, pressing lightly on the inner heel frees the groin.

8. The last thing to keep in mind is that the following exercises might be the beginning sessions of the most important learning you'll ever do. Yoga trains us to become more sensitive; at the same time it re-educates our muscles so that they can more easily hold us erect and move us through the gravitational field. Because there's often an inverse relationship between sensitivity and force, the last caveat is the most important. When working with the material in this chapter, remember to pay attention to subtlety of sensation. Don't be tempted to overexert. Instead, work effortlessly to discover the beautiful truth that "less is more."

In mechanics and in exercise physiology, weight transfer is often referred to as "load bearing." In regard to bearing the load of our body within earth's gravitational field, the pelvic and shoulder girdles are pivotal. The loads they bear and the weight they transfer must be balanced front-to-back and side-to-side or structural difficulties ensue. For example, a tight psoas on the left side of the body may create an uneven pelvic tilt that puts undue pressure on the lower right sacrum, causing pain in that quadrant. This in turn has other implications for the legs and feet and may create a slight scoliosis in the spine as well as some misalignment in the shoulders.

In a perfect world, we would all be perfectly balanced: we would be ambidextrous, both sets of toes would point forward when we stand, and both right and left biceps would be the same size. We don't, however, live in a perfect world. Because of the work we do, the kinds of physical conditioning we're taught and the genetic predispositions we've inherited we have all developed some funny ways about us. We stand on one foot more than the other. We slump forward with bellies protruding or are so bound up in our hamstrings that our buttocks create mini shelves that stick out behind. One of the effects of our yoga practice is the amelioration of both inherited and learned asymmetries.   Because of their importance to weight bearing and movement, bringing balance to the hip and shoulder girdles is foundational; learning to work with each becomes a study in fundamental principles of alignment, weight bearing and movement.

The Pelvic Girdle, Legs and Feet

A cross between a saddle and a leaky bowl, the pelvis transfers body weight from the trunk and arms to the legs, feet and ground.   Rather than being one piece as we may think, the bony structure of the pelvis is formed by two halves, the back and front of which are wed by two of the most interesting and fragile joints in the body. Each half of the pelvis mirrors the other and is comprised of 3 fused bones, the ileum, the ischium and the pubis. The ileum, the largest of the three, transfers weight from the trunk and arms to the spine and legs through the sacrum, a triangularly shaped structure that includes the tailbone. The sitz bones (*ischial tuberosities*) form the lowest part of the ischium to become the weight-bearing points of contact between our bodies and whatever surface we're sitting on.

The pubis joins the ischium toward the front of the body. Here the bones are loosely fitted one to the other with a thin piece of gelatinous cartilage between them. This soft connective tissue allows a small amount of play in the front of the pelvis. This play, as any good bridge builder will tell you, is a way of maintaining needed flexibility within supporting structures in order to prevent cracking under sudden shifts in weight distribution. At the back of the body, the two halves of the pelvic bowl join at the sacrum, a series of fused vertebrae that fan triangularly to a point, which is the tailbone. The sides of the triangle

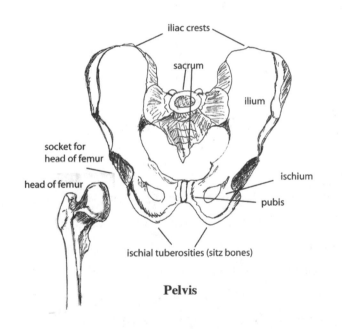

Pelvis

are fluted, not straight, as one might expect. Similarly, the edges of each half of the ilia are also fluted, each curve fitting neatly into a corresponding but oppositely curved portion of the sacrum.   The resultant sacro-iliac (SI) structure is held together by the articulation between the mutually irregular surfaces and by ligaments, which keep the surfaces from slipping along this fault-line joint.

In building construction, the process of fusing support elements is called "joinery." Skilled joinery is an art that combines aesthetics with sound engineering to create stability and elegance. In the body, the fusion of the 2 halves of the pelvis within the SI is an example of joinery in its most elegant form. The curvilinear surfaces at the interface optimize the transfer of weight from the trunk to the legs through the pelvis. In mechanical terms, this means that the joint is "loaded" so that force is distributed over the greatest surface area possible in order to diffuse the effects and minimize the impact at any given point. It's a kind of bio-mechanical democracy, if you will, that allows the sacrum to withstand the physical stresses of standing erect in a gravitational field over an extended period of time—say a life.

While the SI joint is sublime, it's not necessarily stable in all of us. Despite the fact that curves on the ilium often fit neatly into the periphery of the sacrum, the SI joint is prone to displacement. Its instability stems from the very feature that makes it so good at dispersing weight: surfaces articulate, but none is imbedded within another. In addition, the sacrum is subject to myriad forms of misalignment that result from unevenly developed musculature, habitually favoring one leg over the other and injury. Further, the iliopsoas, the primary stabilizing muscle, is often more contracted on one side than on the other. Attached to the lumbar spine on one end and to the inner edge of the thighbone at the other, a tight psoas can be responsible for lower back pain, uneven hips and compromised range of motion.

Set within the circular openings at each side of the pelvis, the ends of the femur (thigh) bones form one part of a joint in which one structure *is* embedded within another. This ball and socket joint allows range of motion in 6 directions: flexion (when the body and leg move towards each other), extension (when the leg and torso move away from each other), abduction (legs move apart), adduction (legs move together), internal (also called medial) rotation and external (also known as lateral) rotation.

Because it houses the reproductive organs and the intestines, from which nutrients are absorbed, the pelvic bowl, particularly in the vicinity of the lower abdomen, is the seat of untold personal power and energy. And because pelvic stability and symmetry are essential to posture, balance and optimal range of motion, we'll be directing our attention first to the kinds of exercises that foster these qualities; that is, we'll be working with the adductors, the muscles of the inner thighs and with the illiopsoas. The psoas passes through the core of this power center; the inner thighs draw us into it. For these reasons, the adductors play a vital role in fostering both strength and balance.

Paradoxically, these are some of the most underused muscles in our bodies. Furthermore, understanding how they function is crucial to understanding many of the actions of the most

42

common standing poses; mountain, any of the lunges, chair, warrior 1, head-to-knee pose, revolved triangle and warrior 3 all require considerable strength and dexterity in the adductors. The following series aims to awaken the inner thighs, to stabilize the pelvis and to release tension in the psoas.

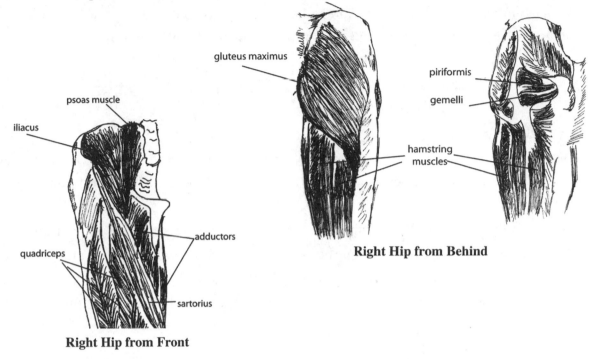

Right Hip from Behind

Right Hip from Front

PELVIC STABILIZATION AND SPINAL EXTENSION

Purpose: To promote pelvic stability and leveling as well as spinal lengthening through "loading," i.e., weight bearing and transfer. Because the weight of the thighs is directly over the hips, it acts as a gentle downward pressure to even the sacrum and from there to distribute the vertebrae evenly along the spine. Alignment thus moves like a gentle wave from the hips to the shoulders and neck.

- Lie on your back with your knees bent and your feet at the wall, making sure your knees are directly over your hips. Both knee and hip joints form 90 ° angles. Keep your feet hip distance apart.

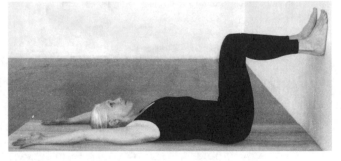

- Reach your arms beyond your head, rotating them so your palms face up. Arrange your shoulder blades so that they make equal contact with the floor.

- Notice the weight at your sacrum/lumbar spine. Breath deeply, from your lower abdomen to your throat.
- Allow your lumbar spine to release and adjust your hips so that both sides of your sacrum are equally engaged with the floor. One way to do this is to work from your lower abdominal muscles and your psoas, drawing these in and down toward your back.
- Hold for 30 seconds to 5 minutes.

KNEE SQUEEZE

Purpose: Pelvic stabilization through the engagement of the adductors (inner thighs). The actions in this simple exercise are essential for poses such as chair/utkatasana and squat/malasana.

- Begin lying on your back with your feet on the wall, your knees above your hips and your arms reaching beyond your head, palms up. Make wall contact with your inner and outer heels and the balls of the big and little toes.
- Create resistance by placing a yoga block, a blanket/mat roll or a small pillow between your knees.
- As you exhale, draw your knees towards each other, gently squeezing the block or pillow.

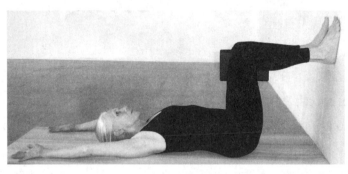

- As you inhale, release the squeeze only enough to relax your inner thighs/adductors without letting go of the block/pillow.
- Repeat 6-10 times.

PELVIC TILT

Purpose: To explore the range of motion in the pelvis; to engage and release the psoas; to find a comfortable supine working position for the lumbar spine and sacrum.

- Begin lying on your back, with your feet against the wall and your knees directly over your hips. Your shins will be parallel to the earth.
- As you inhale, tilt the top of your pelvis towards the wall, pressing your tailbone t

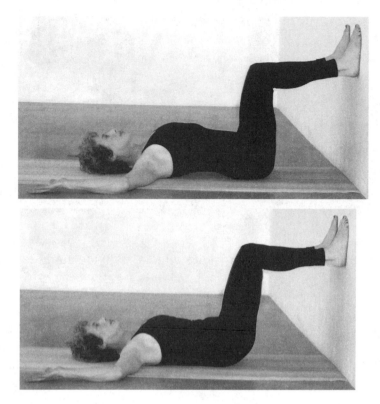

towards the earth. Your lumbar spine will rise up, accentuating its natural curve.

• As you exhale, inflate your lumbar spine, tilt your tailbone up until your lower back comes to the floor. Feel your sacrum widen.

• Inhale, and arch slightly. Exhale, tilt.

• Continue for 3-5 more breaths.

• When you finish, take a few breaths with your spine neutral. *Note: for added muscular engagement, this can be done with resistance between the knees.*

PELVIC LIFT

Purpose: To relax the psoas and awaken the back body; to explore the relationships among the feet, legs, abdominals and spinal muscles; to create both a mechanical expansion of the thoracic cavity/ribcage and an energetic movement from the pelvis to the throat; to strengthen the neck and release tension in the shoulders; to massage the spine and stimulate the kidneys. It also prepares the neck and shoulders for bridge, plow, and shoulderstand.

• Lie on the floor with your sitz bones and the backs of your legs against the wall. Your arms are resting next to your body, palms down.

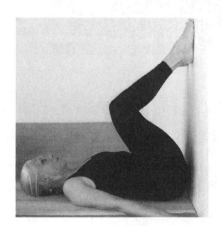

• As you exhale, bend your knees, pressing the soles of your feet against the wall. Engage your inner heels first, then the balls of your big and little toes. Distribute pressure evenly across the arches of both feet. Tilt your tailbone up. Feel your lumbar spine expand and make light contact with the floor.

• Inhale, lower your tailbone.

• Exhale again, raising your tailbone a little higher, feeling the muscles along your lower back ribs—the area around your kidneys—expand as they come in contact with the floor.

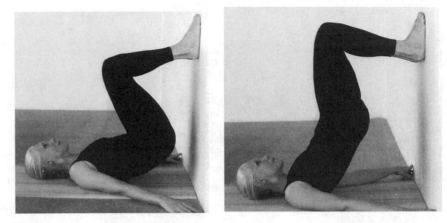

- Inhale, lower your tailbone and tilt your pelvis.
- Exhale again, raising your tailbone even higher, so that you feel your shoulder blades engage with the earth.
- Inhale, lowering your tailbone. Tilt your pelvis.
- Continue to lift and lower for up to a minute, feeling both an expansion of your chest wall on the in-breath and an energetic flow from your pelvis to your throat. Move in sync with the rhythm of your breath, observing sensations

Note: The pelvic lift can be done with resistance--a yoga block or pillow--between the knees.

PSOAS RELEASE / BRIDGE

Purpose: To stretch the psoas, strengthen the thighs and neck; to explore the relationships between the feet, knees, hips, inner thighs and inner belly. This pose uses the wall for orientation instead of for support or resistance. To increase awareness, place a block or blanket roll between your knees.

- Begin on your back with your knees bent and your feet flat on the floor, hip distance apart. The outer edges of your feet are parallel and your toes point towards the wall in front of you.

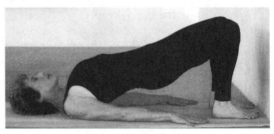

- Press inner and outer heels and the balls of the big and little toes into the floor; press your knees and shins away from your head as if you're trying to reach the wall with them.
- Keeping your buttocks muscles relaxed, lift your hips on an inhale.
- EITHER hold the pose for 4-8 breaths or work dynamically, lifting and lowering 4-8 times.
- Do the same with your buttocks' muscles tightened and notice the difference in effect.
  Note: If you have sacral issues, do not follow this suggestion.

46

The adductors help us "hug to midline" when we sit, stand, walk and do our yoga. The abductors, on the other hand, open our legs to the sides. The following pose involves the gluteus. piriformis and gemelli muscles of the buttocks to widen the angle between the legs and to alleviate tension in the outer hip. A not-so-secondary effect is that it also stretches the inner thighs; thus it becomes a counter pose to those that strengthen these muscles. There are 2 variations: 1 that utilizes gravity and 1 that engages the muscles.

WIDE ANGLE VARIATION 1

Purpose: to cultivate range of motion in the hip and stretch the adductors as well as the connective tissues deep within the hip; to ameliorate tension in the outer hip and lower back.

- Lie on your back with your legs up the wall so that your ankles and knees are directly over your hips. Your arms are at your sides, palms down, or rest your hands on your thighs.
- Open your legs to the sides as far as they'll comfortably go. Breathe deeply and allow yourself to relax. Let gravity do the work here.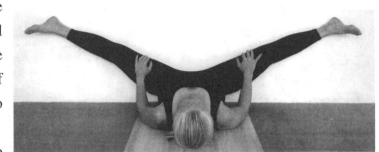
- Allow your thighs to rotate externally and your toes to open to the sides if they do so, but encourage both sides of your sacrum to remain equally in contact with the floor.
- Hold for 30 seconds or up to 5 minutes. As you hold the pose, you'll feel your inner thighs release incrementally, and you may need to readjust your hips and lower back. Be careful not to overstretch. When the pose becomes uncomfortable, come out of it.

WIDE ANGLE VARIATION 2

Purpose: To stretch the adductors and increase range of motion in the hip. In this variation, your legs may not open as far, but active calves and thighs afford resistance, which encourages a greater stretch in the body of the muscle. In addition, muscular engagement precludes connective tissue involvement, thereby preventing injury in the groins from overstretching. This prepares the legs for both seated and standing wide legged forward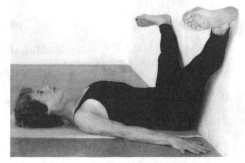

bends.

- Lie on your back as above, BUT press your sitz bones gently against the wall, anchor your heels at the wall as well, and flex your toes towards your knees. Rotate your inner thighs towards the wall.
- Tilt your pelvis so that the top moves towards the wall and your lower back retains its natural curve.
- Hold for 6-10 breaths.

ASYMMETRICAL WIDE ANGLE POSE

If you're very tight or working with someone who is or if your focus is on maintaining pelvic integrity while learning to open the inner thighs, use the following variation. The legs in this pose have a similar shape to the legs in the standing balance, half moon. For this reason, it can be considered a preparatory pose for this foundational standing balance asana.

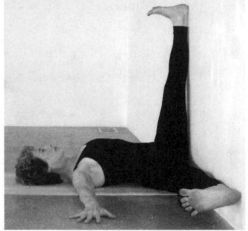

- Anchor your left heel at the wall by pressing on it lightly.
- Place your hands on the floor, palms down, and encourage both sides of your lower back to rest equally against the floor.
- Release your right leg towards the floor, slowly sliding your heel down the wall until you feel your left hip rise.
- Move the left hip back to the floor and hold the pose, activating your right leg by pressing your heel lightly into the wall and rotating your inner thigh to the wall as well.
- Hold for 6-10 breaths.
- Inhale your right leg back up the wall, and repeat the pose on the other side.

Flexion, through which the angle between the trunk and the legs is diminished, is the most common movement of the hip. We move our legs towards our torsos when we walk, when we drive and when we sit to eat or work at our desks. When we bend over to pick up a child or a piece of cake that fell on the floor, we bring our ribs towards our legs. This, too, is an example of flexion. Because forward bending is so familiar to our bodies, many yoga programs begin with flexion and work through the movements of the hips from there. In fact, each of the exercises described thus far utilizes flexion.

Besides familiarity, forward bending often has the added advantage of stretching the hamstrings, which are characteristically tight in many people. Although we don't think of them as forward bends, the preceding poses as well as the supine postures that follow make use of flexion to release the lower back. But, before we look at the exercises, let's talk about feet.

When we stand, our feet are the points of contact between ourselves and the earth. For many of us, however, the quality of that contact is much inhibited. Irregularities such as bunions, heal spurs, plantar fasciatis and fallen arches shift our weight to the left or right, forward or back. The resultant foot print, were we to be standing in sand, shows too much pressure in some places and too little in others. This uneven distribution of weight across the 3 arches and 26 bones of our feet can be addressed in non-weight bearing poses.

The following exercise is done in a supine position with our feet against a wall to help us understand and modify our habits of turning out or in at the ankles or pressing too hard in one area of the foot and too little in another. In addition, it helps us appreciate how alignment of the foot affects our knees and hips as well as our calves, hamstrings, quadriceps, hip flexors and gluteus muscles. While lying on our backs, we can more readily set patterns for right relationships among our muscles and joints than if we were exploring the same alignment while also bearing the weight of our bodies.

SUPINE FOOT PRESS

Purpose: To become aware of the sole of the foot and its points of contact; to explore the ways in which the points of contact affect the ankles, knees and hips. This single leg extension also begins teaching the body to understand the role the straight leg plays in anchoring the pelvis in reclining hand to foot pose and its variations.

- Lie on your back with your left knee bent, your right knee straight and the sole of your right foot at the wall. Anchor your pelvis by tilting it slightly forward and making sure that both sides of your sacrum make equal contact with the floor.
- Press your inner heel against the wall. You may feel your calf press against the floor as well as your hamstrings. See if you can also feel your quadriceps engage and your right groin hollow slightly.
- Hold your leg in this position for 5-7 breaths.
- Bend your knee slightly so that your heel comes off the baseboard and your toes flex.

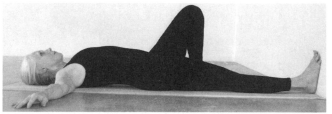

- Hugging the wall with the toe pads, gently straighten your toes until the base of each meets the wall. Distribute the contact evenly among all of your toes, from the big to the little, and spread your toes apart, creating as much space between each as you can. Resist the tendency for your knee to roll to the right. Keep your ankle, knee and hip tracking in a single plane.

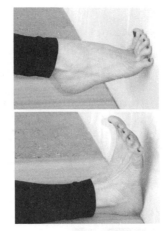

- Keeping your toes spread, straighten your knee until your heel comes back to the wall. Gently flex your foot so that your toes come off the wall.

- Finally, breathe your foot evenly to the wall—front to back, side to side. Extend one last time from your hip, feel your right groin stretch and hollow. Breathe into and through your leg. Hold for 5-7 breaths.

- Repeat the same procedures on your left leg.

RECLINING MOUNTAIN

Purpose: to become aware of spinal alignment from the hips through the shoulders and into the neck and head. To feel the points of contact with the earth and observe what muscles must engage in order to create and maintain the natural curvature of the spine. To prepare for mountain.

- Bring both feet to the wall, hip distance apart. Anchor them so that you're making even contact, side-to-side and front-to-back.

- Draw your shins isometrically towards each other, press your inner thighs down, spread your sitz bones slightly, and move your pelvis until you feel the lumbar spine lift slightly off the floor.

- Press the backs of your hands lightly into the floor while you draw your shoulder blades towards each other. Gently press the back of your head down to release your neck and open your throat. Hold 5-7 breaths.

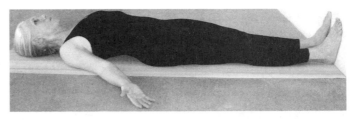

- Raise your arms up and back, lowering them to the floor beyond your head.

- Keeping your abdominals relaxed, draw your shoulder blades lightly 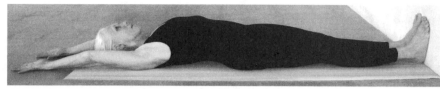 toward each other, lifting your chest and sternum as you do so. Allow your thoracic spine to settle back into the floor.
- Lift and lower your chin to release your neck; press lightly against the occiput, the rounded portion of the back of your head.
- Take 5-7 breaths.

ASYMMETRICAL LEG FLEXION

Purpose: To explore the role of the inner heel and the adductors in promoting pelvic stability; to promote tracking of the leg joints during flexion; to initiate a stretch in the hamstrings; to cultivate an understanding of the way in which the engagement of paired muscles enhances stretching.

- Lie on your back with both feet against the wall and your knees straight. Your arms are at your sides.
- Raise your right leg, bending your knee to 90°. Keep your knee over your hip and take hold of your right thigh with both hands. Press your thigh into your hands as you resist this forward movement with equal but opposite energy.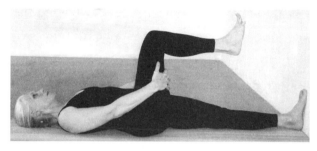
- Draw your shoulder blades towards each other and engage your biceps.
- Tilt your pelvis slightly to maintain the curve in your lower back.
- Notice the tendency for your hips to come off square and, using your left inner heel and inner thigh as well as your psoas, level your hips.
- Variations: point and flex your right foot; rotate the ankle in both directions.
- Take 5-7 breaths. Repeat on other side.

Note: Because of its shape, this pose prepares the hips and legs for extended and supine hand-to-foot pose and their variations as well as for all forms of crescent warrior.

GROIN RELEASE

Purpose: To stretch the groins and release the psoas and lower back. This pose further encourages pelvic stability through anchoring the inner straight leg. There are 2 versions: (A) in which the leg resists the forward pull of the arms and (B) in which the quadriceps muscles are relaxed. Each does slightly different things.

A. **Purpose**: To bring stability to the pelvis through isometric contraction and psoas release.

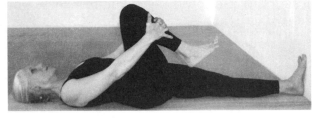

- Begin lying on your back with your knees straight and the backs of your legs against the floor. Adjust your weight so that both shoulder blades make equal contact with the floor. Breathe deeply and evenly.

- On an exhale, bend your right knee and draw your thigh towards your right ribs. Bring your hands to your shin, pressing them against your leg and your leg against your hands. If your hands don't easily circle your shins, use a strap. Thread the strap behind your thigh and, using both hands, draw the strap towards your chest as you press your leg away.

- Press your left inner heel into the wall. Keeping this contact consistent, move some energy into your big toe as well and then distribute it to the outer edges of your foot. Keep the top of your pelvis tilting towards the wall in order to maintain the natural lumbar curve.

- Keep your left inner thigh rotating down.

- Hold for 5-7 breaths. Release and switch sides.

B. **Purpose**: to promote full flexion of the hip joint; to release the adductors where they attach at the pubis; to release the lower back, the piriformis and the gluteals.

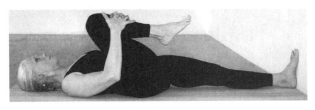

- Lie on your back as shown above, keeping shoulders and pelvis aligned.

- On an exhale, bend your right knee and draw it towards your ribs.

- Slide your hands towards your foot until they make contact with your shin midway between your knee and your foot.

- Without resisting the forward press of your arms, draw your thigh as close to your chest as it will go. Allow your lumbar curve to disappear, but be mindful of your lower back.

52

- Maintain energy in your left leg, pressing through the inner heel towards the wall, keeping your inner thigh rotating toward the floor.
- Hold for 5-7 breaths.
- Inhale to release and exhale to the other side.

Extension is generally defined as the straightening of a joint. Relaxed extension is also known as anatomical position, which, for the hip, occurs when we stand with our knees and ankles tracking below our hips and shoulders. Extension also takes the leg toward the back plane of the body, shortening the angle between it and the trunk, as when we walk or run. The primary muscles responsible for this movement are the hamstrings and gluteus maximus.

Lying straight-legged on our backs creates relaxed extension. To bring the leg beyond the plane of the trunk, we must rise to our hands and knees.

SIMPLE LEG EXTENSION

Purpose: to promote extension of the hip; to explore the relationships among hip, knee, ankle and toes; to stretch the hamstrings and foster joint mobility.

Note: technically, this pose demonstrates flexion because the angle between the front of the leg and the torso is smaller than the angle between the back of the leg and the spine. However, it preps the lower back and legs for leg lifting and for back bending, in which the legs are brought behind the torso.

- Begin on your hands and knees close enough to the wall that you can touch the baseboard with your toes when you straighten your knee but far enough away that your knee becomes as straight as your hamstrings will allow.
- Straighten your right leg behind you.
- Turn your toes under and press them lightly against the floor; press the balls of your toes against the wall.

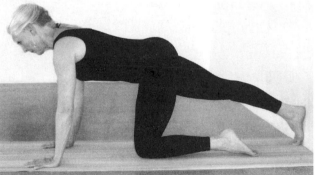

- Level your hips.
- Press your foot back as if you're trying to dislodge your thigh from your hip. Notice the effect on your knee, groins, and hip.
- Draw your thigh back into its socket and notice the sensations and the effects on your hip and leg.

- Find anatomical neutral for you (i.e., the place that feels "just right") and hold the position for 4-6 breaths.
- Change sides.

Note: Any extension of the leg, even this simple reaching back, has an element of backbending to it. The following pose engages not only the leg muscles but also those of the lower spine.

LEG LIFT

Purpose: to stretch the groins, hamstrings, hip flexors; to strengthen the lower back; to explore the relationships among pelvis, legs and feet.

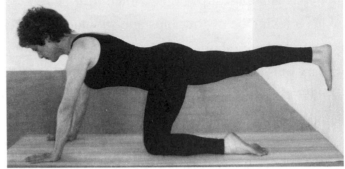

- Begin on your hands and knees close enough to the wall that you can place your foot on the wall (hip height) when you straighten your knee but far enough away that your knee becomes as straight as your hamstrings will allow.
- Raise your right leg behind you and press your foot into the wall.
- Turn your toes so they point down and press lightly and evenly against all points of contact. Make even contact, front-to-back and side-to-side.
- Draw your right hip down so that it's level with the left, and soften your knee without bending it.
- Notice your lower back; if it's sagging, tilt the bottom of your pelvis forward until you remove the excess curvature.
- Hold for 4-6 breaths.
- Change sides.

Of all the movements of the hip, internal and external rotation are the most difficult to visualize. This is, in part, because of the multiple layers of muscle and connective tissue that surround the joint wherein the head of the femur is embedded within its socket. External rotation draws the inseam of the leg towards the sky. When we're lying down, this will turn the toes out. Internal rotation, on the other hand, points the thigh in and down and the toes towards each other. Most of us are disposed by genetics and conditioning to do more one than the other. We stand with toes turned out or in, with our weight pressing towards the outer or inner edges of our feet and with our ankles turning this way and that. Since what happens at the hips affects the rest of the body, cultivating balance through increasing our range of external and internal

54

rotation is essential, especially as we age. The muscles responsible for adduction, abduction, flexion and extension combine to perform these complex movements that keep us young and off the surgeon's table. What follow are 3 versions of classic hip opening to encourage external rotation and 2 exercises that cultivate a spiraling movement of the thigh inward.

HIP OPENER 1

Purpose: To increase range of motion in the hip; to foster awareness of pelvic alignment within asymmetry; to teach the hip the shape necessary for more advanced external rotations, pigeon, half bound lotus forward bend, fire log and lotus being the most notable.

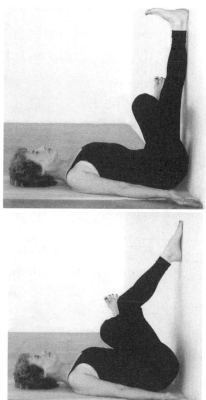

- Begin lying on your back with your sitz bones and the backs of your legs in contact with the wall.
- Bend your right knee, and place your right ankle on your left thigh, just below (towards your torso) your left knee. Flex your right toes towards your shin and lightly press your right knee toward the wall.
- Keep your left heel and inner thigh and sitz bone in contact with the wall; using your psoas and your lower abdominals, level your hips so that both sides of your lower back make equal contact with the floor.
- Take several deep breaths, and, if you need more "juice" in your right hip, bend your left knee, sliding your heel down the wall until the traction in your right hip feels adequate.
- Take note of the tailbone. It will want to come up; resist this upward movement. Keep both legs active, working with resistance, one to the other.
- Hold for 4-10 breaths or up to a minute and switch sides.

HIP OPENER 2

Purpose: Same as above, but the focus here is on maintaining pelvic stability within the stretch. (photo next page)

- Begin lying on your back with your feet on the wall. Your knees, which are over your hips, form an "L."
- Press lightly on your left inner heel and the ball of the left big toe as you bend your

right knee, placing your ankle on your left thigh just below (towards your body) your knee.

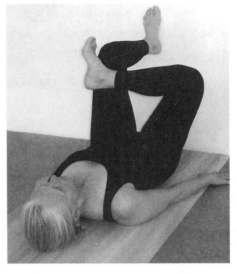

- Flex your right toes towards your shin and use your right hand to encourage your knee to move towards the wall. As you do this, draw your left hip towards the earth by engaging the psoas and adductors to keep your pelvis stable and level. This counteracts the tendency of your weight to shift to the right.
- Engage the adductors of your left leg as well as your quads. Even though your left foot makes active contact with the wall, there's a slight head-ward pressure at the thighbone that creates resistance at the right ankle.
- Take 4-6 breaths and change sides.

BOUND ANGLE / BUTTERFLY

Purpose: To promote a symmetrical increase in range of motion while maintaining pelvic stability and alignment.   As in the wide angle pose, this pose can be passive or it can actively engage the muscles of the legs.   Variations in the actions are illustrated in the photos.

- Lie on your back with your legs up the wall.
- On an exhale, bend both knees, bringing both feet to the wall and sliding them towards your torso as far as is comfortable.
- Open your knees to the sides, bringing the soles of your feet together.

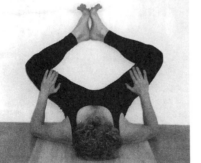 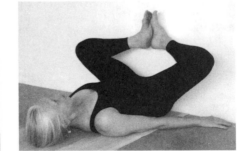

For a <u>passive stretch</u>, allow your feet to open as they will. Hold up to a minute.

For an <u>active stretch</u>, place your hands on your thighs and press your legs lightly towards the wall. Press the outer edges of your feet together, and if possible, also keep your heels and the balls of your big toes together. This recruits your adductors and quads.   Hold 5-7 breaths.

56

EAGLE LEGS

Purpose: To decompress the sacrum through internal rotation of the femur; to promote range of motion in the hip joint. This exercise also prepares the hips and legs for garudhasana, eagle pose. There are 2 versions: 1 with your knees making an "L" and 1 with your sitz bones at the wall.

Knees at 90°

- Begin lying on your back with both feet on the wall, hip distance apart. Align your knees so that your shin and thigh bones are perpendicular to each other.
- Keeping the 90° bend in your knee, raise your foot from the wall and draw your shin towards you. Cross your right thigh over your left so that your knees fit snuggly, one to the other.

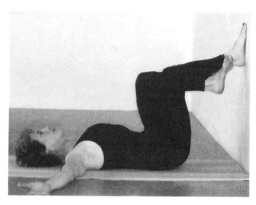

- Press the outer edge of your right shin against the outer edge of your left shin; return the pressure with your left shin pressing into the right equally, or slide your right foot under your left calf.
- Maintain resistance in your psoas and core so that your right hip stays in contact with the floor. The contact should be equal to that of your left hip. Against this downward movement of your hip, rotate the femur further inward by pressing a little harder on your right lower leg.
- Hold 5-7 breaths and change legs.

Sitz Bones at the Wall

- Begin lying on your back with the backs of your legs against the wall and your arm in any comfortable position.
- Bend your right knee, drawing it towards your torso.
- Cross your right leg over the left and hug the outer edges of your lower legs toward each other. If you can, tuck your right foot under the left calf.
- Hold 5-7 breaths and change legs.

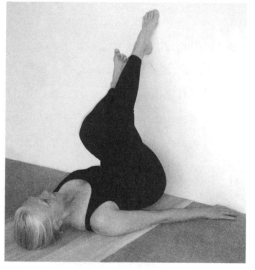

Shoulder Girdle, Arms and Hands

Whereas the pelvis bears and transfers weight from the trunk to the legs and feet, the shoulder girdle bears and transfers the weight of that which we hold and carry to the trunk. The pelvis keeps us grounded; the shoulders enable us to interact with other people and with our surroundings. Because of this, the shoulders are more mobile than the hips and infinitely more complex.

The shoulder girdle is comprised of 4 bones: 2 clavicles (collar bones) and 2 scapulae (shoulder blades), which form an open-ended ring at the top of the torso. The clavicles sit neatly in saddle-like depressions of the manubrium, a quadrangular segment of the upper sternum.

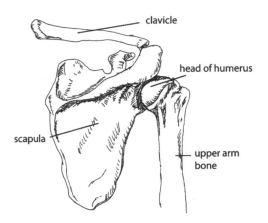

Right Shoulder from Behind

The shape of this articulation allows each collarbone to hinge up and down as its corresponding arm is raised and lowered. It's interesting to note that this is the only place at which the shoulder girdle is connected to the trunk. At the other end of its slight s-curve, each clavicle nestles into a curved edge of one of the shoulder blades. Because our arms require extreme mobility, the scapulae float atop the upper back ribs.

Wrapped in layers of muscle and connective tissues, they're able to move up and down and side-to-side; thus these triangularly shaped bones increase the range of motion in our arms. The head of the upper arm bone is less embedded within its socket than the head of the thigh is within the hip. Instead of being encapsulated, the ball of the humerus rolls along the shallow surface of its socket at the upper edge of the shoulder blade. This depression is edged with cartilage that adheres to both the edge of the blade and to the ball of the upper arm, sealing the joint much as a washer does.

From the saddles at the sternum to the floating scapulae, the joints that form the shoulder girdle are designed to move. But mobility comes at a price. The bones and their articulations with one another sit close to the body's surface and are thus easily dislocated. In addition, the way we live our lives—arms continually reaching forward—brings strain to muscle and connective tissues. For these reasons, getting to know our shoulders is an important first step in using them safely and without injury—both on and off our yoga mats. As with the hips, increasing range of motion within the framework of stability is an objective.

Like the hips, the shoulder blades move in 6 primary ways. For example, the scapulae lift and lower. They also protract, that is they move toward the outer edges of the torso and forward. They retract, i.e., towards the spine. And they rotate in two directions: the lower edges move both towards and away from the spinal column.

From their resting position at the sides of the body, the long bones of the upper arms flex (move forward and up), extend (move back and up), abduct (move up from the side), and adduct (move toward the body after being lifted to the side). Adduction combines with extension to move the arm behind the back and with flexion to move it in front of the body. The upper arm bones also rotate forward and back; rotations combine with each of the other actions to facilitate touching anything within an arm's radius of us.

At the extremes of their range, the movements of the arms affect the ribs and thoracic spine. Furthermore, the movements of the shoulder blades combine with those of the upper arm bones to increase mobility in the shoulders as when the blades lift to assist us in moving our arms above our shoulders and towards our heads. More importantly for our yoga practice, the scapulae can be used as levering agents to resist the movements of the arms. This resistance adds stability to the shoulder gircle and increases both the strengthening and stretching capacity of each pose.

In the following, non-weight-bearing exercises, this objective as well as the cultivation of symmetry within the shoulder girdle has a profound effect on spinal alignment and on optimal use of the arms and shoulders within the repertoire of yoga asanas currently being taught in hatha yoga classes today.

STATIONARY SPINE SERIES

This series explores the relationships among the shoulder blades, upper arms bones, and elbows; to promote stability in the shoulders. Although lying on the back is depicted, all of the exercises in this series can also be done seated and/or standing with the back against the wall. With the body erect, they lose some of their efficacy in that the pelvic loading that helps align the spine is missing. However, they're still a wonderful tool for understanding how the arms and shoulder blades interact with each other.

A. **Purpose:** Arms abduct; forearms rotate; shoulder blades retract. This explores the effect of movement/force in the upper arms relative to the shoulder blades and as such can be a preparation for chaturanga dandasana. Creates awareness of the actions of the muscles of the upper arms and shoulders.

- Lie on your back, with your feet at the wall as in the basic pelvic stabilization exercise. Your feet are hip distance apart, knees over your hips.

- Your arms are at your sides, palms down.
- Bend your elbows to 90° with your palms facing each other, fingers pointing up.
- Draw the bottoms of your shoulder blades slightly towards each other.
- As you inhale, press down on your upper arm bones; exhale and release; keep your abdominal muscles relaxed. Notice what

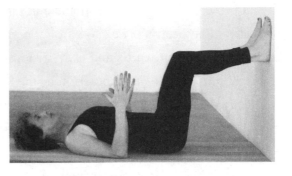

happens to your shoulder blades and to the tips of the shoulders where the collarbone connects.
- Hold this position for several breaths.
- Exhale as you release and repeat 4-6 times.

B. **Purpose:** Arms abduct and rotate; explores protraction and retraction of shoulder blades and the role of the elbows in working with the shoulders; stretches and strengthens the muscles that draw the shoulder blades toward each other on the back.

- Lie on your back as above, feet at the wall, knees over hips, arms in cactus position with your elbows at shoulder height and your forearms perpendicular to your upper arm

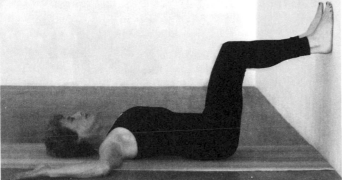

bones, palms up.
- Maintain a 90° bend in your elbows; press the backs of your hands gently to the floor.
- As you exhale, bring your elbows,

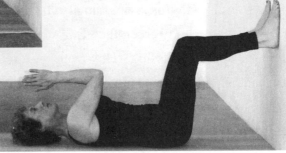

forearms, and palms together above your chest; maintain the 90° bend in your elbows, and resist the tendency of your upper arms to lower towards your body. Feel the backs of your shoulders expand.
- Inhale and open your arms to the floor. Press the backs of your hands towards or into the floor; feel your shoulder blades draw towards each other.
- Repeat the movement 4-6 times.

C. **Purpose:** Explores abduction and adduction of the arm as well as elevation and depression of the shoulder blade; fosters shoulder stability.

- Lie on your back with your feet on the wall.
- Your arms are in cactus position, elbows in line with your shoulders, backs of your hands on the floor, palms facing up.
- As you exhale, glide your hands towards each other along the floor, maintaining the 90° bends in your elbows. Your elbows will slide up as your hands move.
- Inhale while you bring your elbows back to their starting position.
- Exhale; draw your elbows towards your ribs, maintaining the 90° bend.
- Inhale your arms back to their starting position.
- Repeat the movement 4-6 times.

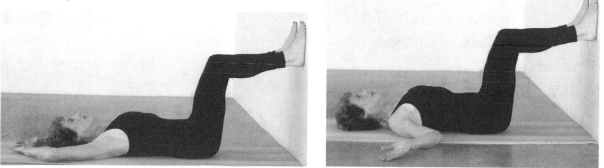

D. **Purpose:** Explores flexion and extension and their effects on the ribs, spine and lower back.

- Begin in the basic pelvic stabilization posture.
- Your arms are next to your body, palms down.
- As you inhale, lift your arms forward, up and then down beyond your head. Your palms will face up when the movement is complete.
- As you exhale, reverse the movement. Press your palms, your forearms and your upper arms into the floor.

•

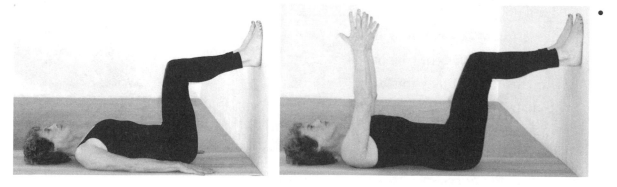

Note the movements of your spine, ribs and pelvis in response to your arms

- Repeat 4-6 times, keeping your pelvis stable as your arms engage your thoracic cavity and lumbar spine.

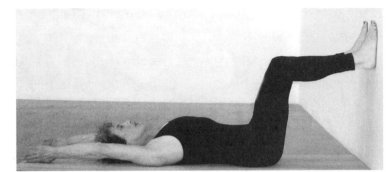

COMBINED ARM RAISE AND PELVIC LIFT

Purpose: Combining the pelvic lift with arm raises is a lovely way to begin a practice. It releases the psoas, gets us in touch with the lower belly, strengthens the neck and encourages spinal awakening. There's a sweet mechanical levering action in the ribcage, contributing to a sense of expansion and increased movement of energy. Some beginning students find the coordination of movements difficult, but with continued practice they're able to enjoy its benefits.

- Begin on your back with your sitz bones at and your legs up the wall. Your arms are next to your sides, palms down.
- Bend your knees and bring your feet to the wall, slightly higher than your hips.
- As you inhale, hug the wall with your feet to engage your calf and quadriceps muscles; engage your abdomen, and begin to lift your hips from the earth.
- Simultaneously, raise your arms until they're vertical and then lower them beyond your head, pressing the backs of your hands into the floor (if they touch).
- Exhale, reversing the direction of movement in both hips and arms.
- Repeat 5-7 times.

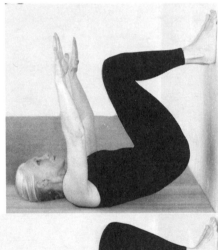

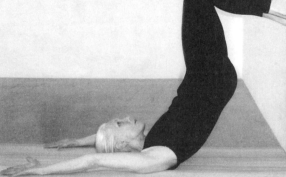

Standing Alignment Basics

When we stand, we put it all together: feet touch the earth on the inner and outer edges equally, and there's even pressure, front to back; the adductors stabilize the pelvis; the lower back maintains its curve; shoulder blades integrate toward the back bone; and the lower abdominals tuck slightly as we raise the chest wall up and away from the navel. Our joints stack neatly from the ankles through the hips to the shoulders so that our weight is evenly distributed throughout the body. It sounds simple enough, but doing it is another matter.
To this end, the following series encourages an appreciation of our standing posture--what it is and what it might become.

MOUNTAIN

Purpose: With our arms at our sides, this is the basic standing pose. It mirrors the spinal alignment exercise done lying on the floor and can be used in conjunction with it to reinforce an understanding of how vertebrea stack and curve. Against the wall we use this pose to explore spinal alignment while standing according to the following principles: femurs back, tailbone rooting, lower back ribs slightly inflated, shoulder blades on the back, ears in line with the shoulders.

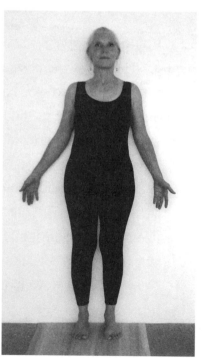

- Stand with your back against the wall, your feet hip-width apart. Tilt the bottom of your pelvis slightly forward and down, but maintain your lumbar curve. Depending on how severe the curve and how much muscle mass you have in your gluteals, your heels will probably not touch the wall. No worries. The point is to keep your hips over your knees and your knees over your ankles.
- Drawing your shoulder blades towards each other, bring your sternum away from your navel. Inhale into the area of your kidneys just underneath your lower back ribs.
- Press the back of your head into the wall as you bring your shoulder blades towards each other.
- Without closing your throat, tuck your chin and gaze forward as if looking at the distant horizon.
- Take 5-7 breaths.

HANDS UP POSE

Purpose: This variation of mountain pose explores spinal alignment with the arms raised.

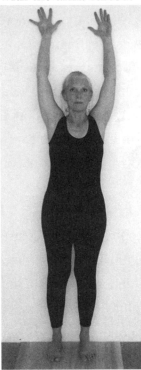

- Begin as above.
- Raise your arms until they become extensions of your torso, hands shoulder width apart. Keeping your elbows straight and the fingers moving up, draw your shoulder blades down your back and towards each other.
- Press the backs of your hands against the wall, draw the lower arms towards each other and externally rotate the upper arms back and away from each other.
- From a stable core, breathe into your arms, opening the meridians that run through the heart to each hand.
- Hold for 5-7 breaths.

Note: this and the previous version of mountain can be combined using movement between them to increase range of motion in the shoulders. Inhale the arms up and exhale them down. All of the static back series of shoulder movements can be performed in mountain as well.

HEEL RAISES

Purpose: The following pose engages the legs, particularly the calves and Achilles tendons to work out kinks in the alignment of the major weight-bearing joints in the body. Ideally, hips stack above knees stack above ankles. Begin in mountain with your back at the wall.

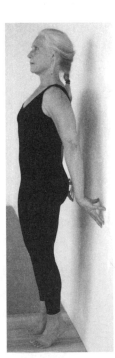

- Your feet are hip distance apart, outer edges parallel, and your weight is evenly distributed side-to-side and front-to-back.
- As you inhale lift your heels off the floor and come onto your toes. Work against any tendency to shift to the inner or outer edges of your feet and keep your hips over your ankles.
- As you exhale, lower your heels to the floor.
- Repeat up to 10 times.

Our hands are an important means of contact with the world outside ourselves. As extensions of our shoulders and arms, they conduct heart energy to that which surrounds us, manipulating things and touching people in an expression of our creativity and feelings. Like our feet, for a myriad reasons, our hands also make uneven contact with the surfaces they touch. Arthritis, carpel tunnel syndrome and tight ligaments render it difficult to spread the fingers and open the palms. A wall cultivates an appreciation for the ways of the hand and its relationship to our wrist, elbow and shoulder. It also assists us in ameliorating the sometimes painful effects of years of neglect.

HANDS AGAINST THE WALL

Purpose: to explore the relationships among the hands, wrists, elbows and shoulders; to align the bones and joints in the arm; to activate internal levers at the wrist and shoulder.

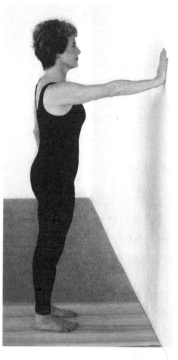

- Begin standing facing the wall, an arm's length away.
- Place your right palm against the wall so that your wrist, elbow and shoulder are at the same height. Your shoulder should be resting in its socket and your elbow as straight as possible.
- Spread your fingers wide, making light contact with the digits and the joints where they meet in the palm. Rotate your hand to the right so that metacarpal of the thumb makes contact with the wall and your pinky finger comes off the wall. Keeping your thumb tacked down, press your little finger into the wall.

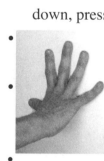 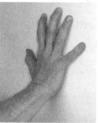

- Raise the heel of your hand, so that your fingers flatten against the wall.
- Lower the heel of your hand and hug this against the wall until the middle of your hand cups inward. Feel your wrist come into a 90° angle.
- Change hands.
- Repeat with both hands, keeping equal effort in both arms and evenly distribute the contact with the surface of the wall throughout the heel of your hands and your fingers.

WRIST RELEASES: WRISTS UP & BACKS OF HANDS AGAINST THE WALL

The following two exercises bend the wrists in unaccustomed ways. For this reason, they stretch and strengthen the hands and forearms and contribute to healthy functioning of the entire arm.

Purpose: Externally rotates forearms to stretch the muscles that flex the hand, including the *flexor retinaculum*, a transverse muscle at the base of the palm; creates space in the front of the wrist where carpal tunnel sufferers experience the most tightening; externally rotates the upper arm to stretch the biceps.

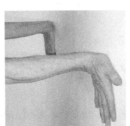

- Stand at the wall, arms at shoulder height, hands at the wall, elbows straight.
- Inhale as you dial your thumbs out as far as they'll comfortably go. Eventually your wrists will do a 180°. Allow your elbows to bend if they do, but stop the rotation at the point where they begin to fold.
- Draw your shoulder blades towards each other and begin to bring your upper and lower arms in alignment with one another by simultaneously pressing the heels of your hands into the wall.
- Spread your fingers as wide as they'll comfortably go, moving some of the energy from the heel of your hand into your fingers. Distribute the pressure evenly across your hand. Be careful not to hyperextend your elbows.
- Take 4-6 breaths.

Purpose: Stretches the extensor muscles of the wrist, hand and lower arm; can be a welcome antidote to computer wrists as well as to any strain brought on by down dog, plank, and handstand.

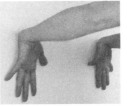

- Stand erect with your arms outstretched, your hands at the wall, your elbows straight and your joints tracking at shoulder height.
- Inhale, bring the backs of your hands to the wall.
- Spread your fingers, and press lightly into the wall.
- At first your elbows might bend to the sides; work to straighten them by drawing your upper arms into the shoulder joints and slightly depressing the blades.
- Hold for 4-7 breaths.

Whether we work against or in conjunction with gravity, aligning our moving parts with one another is essential. We may be able to get by for a little while without employing this fundamental principle of biomechanics, but over time we'll discover that the parts begin to wear. Repair and replacement are poor substitutes for maintaining good working relationships between the trunk and the pelvic and shoulder girdles. In this chapter, we've taken a look at mechanical principles: primarily how the legs are attached to the pelvis and the pelvis to the trunk; the ways in which the movements of the arms and shoulder blades cooperate to bring us optimal range of motion; and the effects of gravity on the spine and limbs. We've also seen how applying a measured force (gravity, muscular effort) can effectively align the lower back and the shoulders and how both the wall and the floor can be used to increase our awareness of our hips, groins and shoulder blades. Touch and loading, then, are important tools for bringing our physical bodies into alignment.

Chapter 4

Taking the Seat: Asana

The posture is firm and soft / sthira-sukham-asanam.

Pajanjali, Sutra II.46

4

The fundamentals of wall work in our yoga practice are simple: resistance increases opening, support increases our sense of well-being and alignment fine-tunes our proprioception. There's another important point to remember, however, when doing the poses--the muscular relationship and energetic connection between the inner thigh (the adductors), the inner edge of the foot (heel and ball of the big toe), the lower abdominal muscles and the sacrum. The combined biomechanical actions of these areas effectively stabilize the pelvis and in so doing create a foundation for the entire body both on and off the mat.

Resistance, both physical and psychological, can become a tool for opening. Simultaneously, both can be obstacles that prevent us from moving beyond where we are. Psychological resistance is often quite subtle; it's hard to determine if not wanting to do something is a result of wisdom, conditioning or the recalcitrance of an inner 2-year old. Physical resistance may take on the same dynamic. The body may resist because of injury or structural limitation, too much weight training and aerobic exercise, or laziness. When we come up against a wall inside ourselves--either psychologically or physically-- we need to decide if there's good reason to heed the warning and work around the block or if we ought to continue on our course and work through what seems to be in the way. One form of physical resistance that may not yield to persistence is the kind of bone-on-bone restriction that inhibits range of motion in a joint. This kind of resistance needs to be worked around because such articulations--whether the result of genetics or injury--often cannot be changed without damage to surrounding tissues or to other joints.

Another form of internal resistance occurs when the ligaments that connect one part of the body to another are tight or when the muscle tissues themselves are inelastic. In this case, if we apply resistance at the other end of the bone, we use the resistance against itself to go beyond the seeming obstacle. An example of this occurs in warrior II when we keep the outer edge of the back foot against the wall as we sink into a lunge with the forward knee. In our asana practice, working with the resistances within the body in conjunction with that of an external wall increases the efficacy of each pose. We get a deeper stretch and more opening as a result.

Support, like resistance, can be both physical and psychological. Physical support is self-evident when we move to the wall for help in one-legged balance poses or in inversions.

But there's a psychological component that's even more important. Many of my students find that they need not actually touch the wall in order to feel less anxious and more stable. Sensing the wall a few inches away from them is enough to give them the confidence they need to relax and enjoy learning how to do a pose. This means they can do it more easily. Security is essential in accomplishing nearly everything we do. The fact that the wall helps us feel secure is one of the major benefits of using it. There is, of course, a danger that we may use this security long after our bodies know how to work without it. But this too, is what yoga's about: learning when it's time to let go.

Although alignment, the third fundamental of wall work, has been discussed in Chapter 3, it bears mentioning that alignment is also multidimensional. It contains physical and energetic aspects. Physically, the wall tells us where we are in space because we can feel it against our shoulder blades, the back of our head, or our heels. So touch is an important way that we use the wall to align our bodies. Another is to use the wall directionally. Aware that it is near us, we aim various body parts (knees in bridge, chest in upward facing bow) towards the wall to get a sense of how to get the most out of an asana. Although energy is in fact a physical property, it's differentiated from touch and direction because it requires a more refined and subtle understanding. Nonetheless, the lines of energy inherent in each asana can be more easily accessed by using the wall as an anchor point from which to stretch. In extended side angle, then, the edge of the back foot becomes the anchor for the sensation of moving energy that occurs as the corresponding arm is stretched forward.

In varying degrees, resistance, support, alignment and pelvic stability all play a role in the following poses. The focus is on maintaining pelvic stability, establishing core awareness and using the wall to emphasize selected key actions in each asana. To this end, the poses are organized into 2 broad categories--Symmetrical and Asymmetrical--based on the pelvis. Symmetrical poses are those in which the legs mirror each other. The classifying principle here is on the role of the adductors, which results in 2 sub groups: that in which the legs are close to or touching each other and that in which the legs are spread. The Asymmetrical category contains those poses in which the legs simultaneously perform differently. The winnowing factor among these postures--internal or external rotation of the back thigh--results in two major sub groups: open and closed hip poses. Of course, no system neatly wraps around each and every case. Because of traditional variations currently being taught, some poses belong in two or more sets. Each of these is presented within the group that best accommodates the primary form of the posture.

In keeping with the organization of the preceding chapter (in which pelvic stability was introduced as a function of inner thigh work), the symmetrical, narrow-legged poses come first, followed by those that abduct, or open, the legs. Within the asymmetrical grouping, the closed hip position will be treated first since they most closely mimic the stabilizing effects of drawing the adductors to mid-line. The last group of poses, those that work asymmetrically with open hips, contains some of the most familiar and most often-taught poses: warrior II, triangle, extended side angle and half moon. They appear toward the end, not because they lack importance as foundational asanas nor because they are more complex than some of the other poses that appear earlier. Rather, they find their place because the configuration of the legs deviates the most from symmetry. The last, very short section contains core cultivation poses. These bridge the classifications. Some are symmetrical and some not. While they are the last poses to be described, they're probably some of the first poses that ought to be learned for without the core, all the rest of the work we do--on and off the mat--tends to fall apart.

You'll note that there are no directions for getting into the poses. Rather, the photos give you the general shape of each. In addition a list of the commonly accepted benefits of each posture, mention of which asana or asanas the wall work prepares us for, containdications as well as a focal point (dristhi) for the eyes are mentioned. These are followed by bulleted lists of key ("Do") and suggested ("Pointers") actions. Variations are depicted in smaller images with key actions described if they're different. One final comment: it's been impossible to include all poses and all variations that can be done at the wall. As a result, you may find that one of your favorites is missing.

Symmetry: Narrow-legged Poses

MOUNTAIN / TADASANA

The first pose in B. K. S. Iyengar's *Light on Yoga*, tadasana, has its analogues in both Ashtanga and in Anusara yogas. Each teaches a slightly different foot position. Whether the entire inner edges of your feet or only your big toes touch will be a matter of preference based on prior training and bone structure. You may also stand with your feet under your hips, which is a more common and anatomically neutral way to stand.

Benefits: aligns the vertebrae, spine and all the major joints in the body; results in good posture and optimal space for internal organs; strengthens ankles; frees the ribs and diaphragm; tones abdominal muscles.

Preparation for: mountain without the wall, all standing poses

Contraindications: none

Drishti: to the horizon, tip of nose

(photo on next page)

Do:

- maintain pelvic stability by engaging your adductors
- tuck the tailbone slightly (unless you have no lumbar curve)
- distribute your weight evenly on and across both feet

Pointers:

- shoulder blades draw towards each other and down the back (notice how this feels against the wall)
- sternum lifts away from navel; ribs telescope up
- chin tucks slightly but throat is open
- lower abdomen draws in

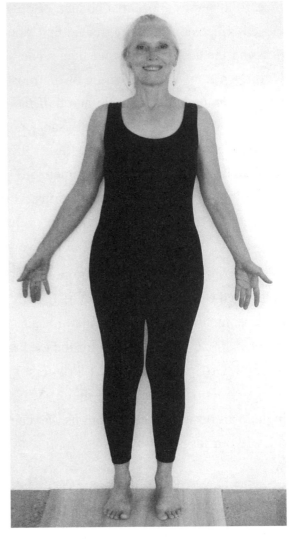

<u>Arms Up</u>

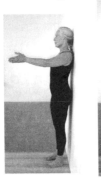

Expands chest wall and ribs to facilitate deepening of the breath.
With arms parallel to floor, draw shoulder blades back towards wall. With arms raised, bring thumbs forward into palms and press the base into the wall

SIDE STRETCH / PARSVOTTANASANA I

Traditionally, parsvottanasana is the name given to side stretching with the torso folded over one leg while the other anchors the body from behind. I've appropriated the Sanskrit here because it most accurately reflects the intent of the following series of poses. Although they stretch the sides of the torso, they can be considered variations of mountain in that the pelvis, legs and feet retain the orientation established in the basic standing pose. The trunk moves in

72

relation to the hips, which remain fixed in order to create the resistance necessary to work the muscles that wrap the ribs--sides, front and back.

Benefits: stretches the hands, arms, and torso; opens the shoulders; isolates muscles and awareness; encourages use of leverage at each end of arm

Preparation for: side bending with and without the wall and in triangle and extended side angle

Contraindications: rotator cuff and other shoulder injuries

Drishti: to the horizon (in variations, up)

Do:

- keep your weight evenly distributed on your feet
- keep your tailbone tucked
- spread your fingers

Pointers:

- fingers reach up
- palm and forearm press into wall
- shoulder blade draws down and in
- opposite shoulder resists upward movement

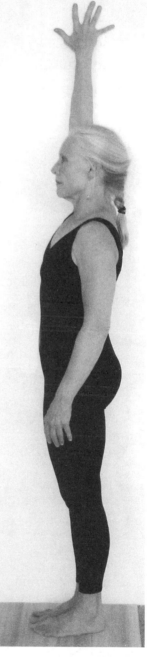

Intense Arm Stretch

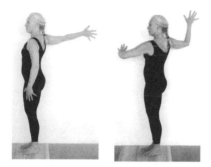

Arm swings back until wrist, elbow, and shoulder are equally distant from the floor. Or elbow bends. Opposite shoulder moves away.

Bending towards Wall

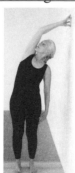

Press fingers into wall.
Maintain even pelvis; telescope ribs up.

Back at Wall

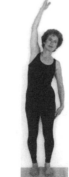

Press shoulder blades into wall.
Maintain even pelvis.

HEART OPENING / ANAHATASANA

"Anahata" is commonly translated as "unstruck." It refers to the idea that love exists by and of itself, not caused by any thing or any one or any specific occasion. The heart opens in love simply because that's what it does.

Benefits: stretches the hands, arms, chest, and torso; opens the shoulders; stretches the psoas; strengthens the postural muscles and lower back; stimulates the thymus gland

Preparation for: back bending, handstand and forearm balance, kneeling anahatasana

Contraindications: neck, shoulder, lower back pain

Drishti: the tip of the nose

Do:
- keep your weight evenly distributed on your feet
- keep your tailbone tucked
- keep your lower abdomen taut

Pointers:

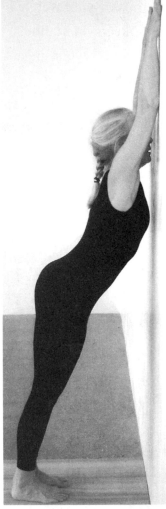

- fingers reach up
- palms and forearms press into wall
- shoulder blades draw down and in
- back of neck remains relaxed; head may turn
- heart moves towards wall

<u>Nose and Toes at Wall</u>
This variation is the starting point for the full pose and is often enough for those with shoulder injuries, tight deltoids and trapezius muscles or for those with lower back and shoulder pain.

In addition to stretching the arms and shoulders, Anahatasana is a valuable backbend, and therefor considered a heart opener.

Cobra and upward facing dog are probably the most well-known of these poses; however sphinx and locust are much more basic in terms of their actions within the body. They target the postural muscles, particularly the lower back by lifting the trunk against active resistance from the legs.

SPHINX AND COBRA / BHUJANGASANA

Technically, "bhujangasana" refers to cobra pose; whereas sphinx is often taught as a preliminary asana, the term is being applied to it here.

Benefits: All versions of sphinx, cobra, and locust alleviate tension in the back and shoulders; strengthen low back and postural muscles; open the chest; stimulate the kidneys and adrenal glands and rejuvenate spine and spirit.

Preparation for: same poses without the wall and for more intense backbends such as upward facing dog, wheel, and bow

Contraindicatioins: rotator cuff and other shoulder injuries, low back pain

Drishti: varies with neck flexibility (tip of nose, third eye, up)

Do:

- press toes or balls of feet and heels into wall to activate legs
- keep tailbone tucked and thighs internally rotating
- keep shoulder blades moving towards each other
- draw sternum forward and then up; avoid compression in lower back

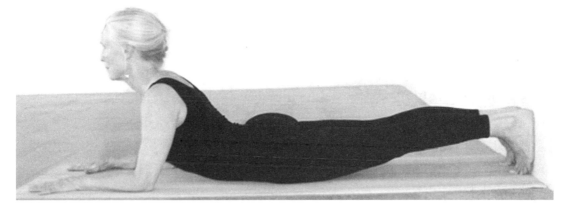

Pointers:

- in sphinx (above), forearms press floor; elbows draw towards ribs
- in cobra variation below, slightly bend elbows; hands move towards feet

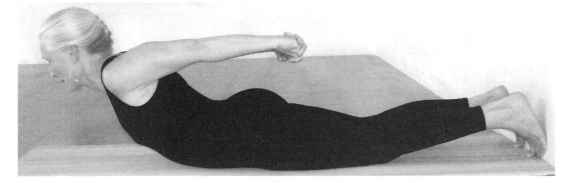

LOCUST / SHALABHASANA

This variation trains nerual pathways as it strengthens the postural muscles.

Pointers:
- thigh bone of the raised leg draws into hip socket
- upper bone of raised arm integrates with the shoulder blade into spine
- lower hand presses into floor and lower foot presses into wall.

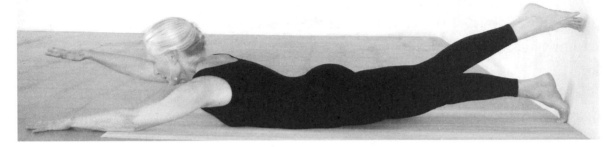

4-LIMBED STAFF / CHATURANGA DANDASANA

This pose, made famous by Ashtanga Vinyasa Yoga, is a major upper arm and core strengthener. It has some of the same actions as tadasana despite the obvious differences in orientation and effort. It also requires (and cultivates) core strength to maintain the natural curvatures of the spine without sagging in the middle or piking the tailbone up. The key, really, is in the feet and legs, which are actively reaching back to keep the torso parallel with the floor.

Benefits: strengthens the arms, wrists, hands and shoulder girdle as well as the core; stretches hamstrings, calves, ankles, Achilles tendons; promotes concentration

Preparation for: same pose away from the wall as well as all arm balances

Contraindications: shoulder, elbow, wrist and hand pain

Drishti: straight ahead

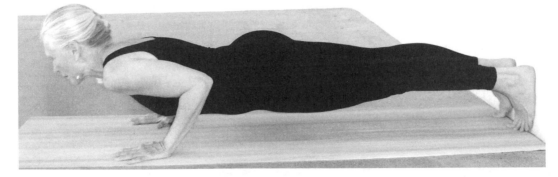

Do:

- press your heels into the wall
- hug your forearms towards each other
- keep your lower abdomen engaged

Pointers:

- thighs rotate internally
- inner arm pits lift
- area of back around kidneys inflates slightly
- shoulder blades move towards each other
- elbows close to ribs

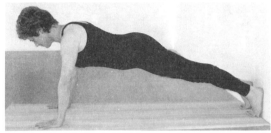

Plank

Shoulders broaden; sitz bones,
and heels form straight line.

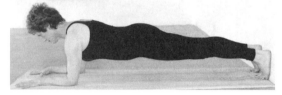

Forearm Plank

Elbows under shoulders, forearms parallel,
shoulder blades on back.

FORWARD BEND / UTTANASANA

Bowing is a universal posture of respect. Taking the gesture further, the standing forward bend eventually brings the head below the heart to signify that what we think is not always so important as how we feel. Decisions that are made with our hearts are more vibrant and long lasting than those made solely with our minds. Notice that there are 2 ways to work a forward bend at the wall. Each has a slightly different intent.

Benefits: stretches the back of the body--primarily the hamstrings and spinal muscles; stimulates blood flow to the brain; calms the nervous system; creates awareness of the back of the legs

Preparation for: forward bending without the wall

Contraindications: sciatica, high blood pressure

Drishti: depends on neck comfort (knees, tip of nose, navel)

Do:
- press sitz bones into wall
- keep weight evenly distributed on both feet and thighs rotating internally
- draw your lower abdomen toward your spine

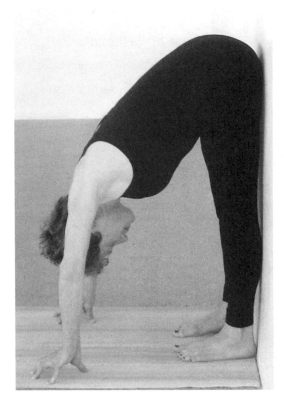

Pointers:
- shoulder blades draw in and towards waist
- neck is relaxed as ears align with shoulders
- spine works towards being straight rather than rounded (making teepees with your hands and staying on your fingers creates length so the thighs can clear the belly

Half Forward Bend

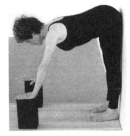

Works legs more than back. Hands press on blocks.

Sitz Bones Resting on Wall / Wall Drape

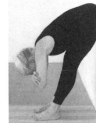

Allow weight to rest on wall. Torso relaxes into gravity. Knees can bend. Hands hold opposite elbows or rest on floor.

Half Wall Drape

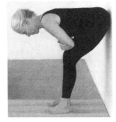

Rest forearms on thighs, tuck tailbone slightly, release neck and head.

Hands under Feet/Wrist Release

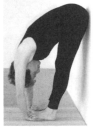

Press balls of toes into hands and hands into feet.

DOWNWARD FACING DOG / ADHO MUKHA SVANASANA

"Dog Pose," as this is affectionately known by those who do it regularly, is one of those asanas about which you wonder, "Why?" at first, then go "Aaaaahhhhhh" when it becomes a familiar friend. Done at the wall, there's an even more delicious sense of opening than usual--and more stability in the legs and pelvis.

Benefits: stretches the entire back side of the body from the heels through the arms; opens the shoulders; strengthens the arms; rests the heart; stimulates digestion

Preparation for: down dog without the wall; hand stand and forearm balance with and without the wall

Contraindications: rotator cuff and other shoulder injuries; high blood pressure; carpal tunnel syndrome, heart disease

Drishti: depends on comfort of neck (navel, legs, nose)

Do:

- press heels into wall
- spread fingers wide and point thumbs towards each other
- maintain tuck in lower abdomen

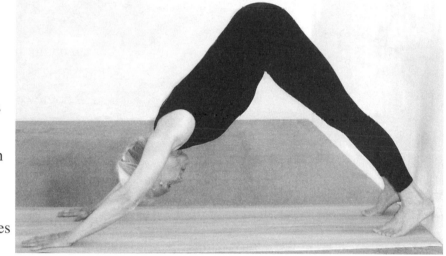

Pointers:

- sitz bones widen
- shoulder blades draw towards each other
- forearms lightly squeeze towards each other
- upper arms lift and rotate externally
- neck releases

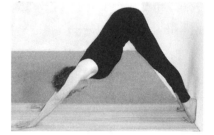

Toes at Wall

Balls of toes press into wall w/heels high to encourage abdominal lift and increased stretch in arms, legs, and spine. Persons with bunions may find this version uncomfortable.

<u>Wall Dog</u>

The benefits of wall dog are many, most importantly, however is that it maintains some of the same shoulder and pelvic actions as down dog but in a non-weight-bearing situation. The hands are slightly higher than the shoulders, and for more shoulder work, the forearms can be placed at the wall instead of the hands. The assist helps teach the body how to use the pelvis and thigh bones to traction the spine, thus increasing the stretch along the back.

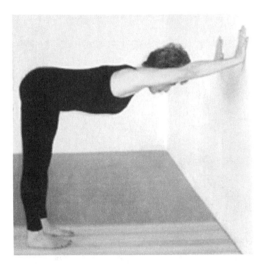

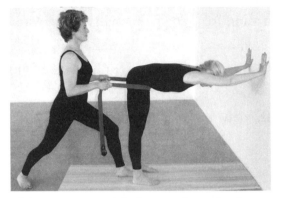

Place strap on hip bones; keep both sides hip width apart & pull straight back so as not to compress the sacrum.

STAFF POSE / DANDASANA

Sitting up straight is a lot harder than it looks. Staff pose, with or without the wall is deceptive in that it doesn't appear that there's much going on. Nonetheless, it encourages good posture, and the actions that create the pose are fundamental to all of the seated asanas: the hamstrings flatten on the floor so that the femurs are firm against the floor; the sitz bones, too, anchor the pelvis as the thighs rotate intenally. Dandasana's cousin, legs up the wall, is considered restorative in that it's usually done without any effort.

Benefits: tones the abdomen, relieves intestinal bloating, expands the chest, activates the meridians on the backs of the legs, cultivates an understanding of working the shoulder blades on the back, tones the kidneys

Preparation for: same pose without the wall; seated forward bend; L handstand

Contraindications: low back pain

Drishti: at the horizon or the tip of the nose

80

Do:

- flex toes and spread them evenly back
- press ankles together and heels away from torso
- tuck chin slightly and press fingers or heels of hands into floor

Pointers:

- shoulder blades flatten and press into wall
- sternum lifts away from navel; lower back curves
- legs together, inner thighs rotate in and down

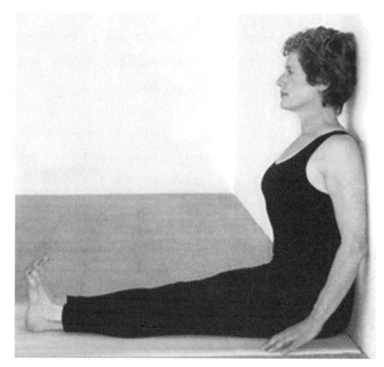

Legs Up the Wall

This pose is included because it bears close resemblance to staff pose. Of course weight is

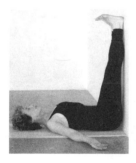

distributed differently, but some of the actions are similar. In *active version* toes flex towards knees, sitz bones press into wall, shoulder blades and back of head press lightly into floor, inner thighs rotate in and back to wall, lower belly draws towards spine. In *passive version* body sinks into floor, muscles relax, weight of legs aligns pelvis and spine. A block or blanket may be inserted beneath the sacrum to increase the effect.

Arms Reach

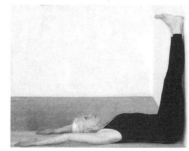

Expands ribs and accentuates lumbar curvature in lower back.

Getting There

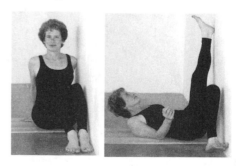

HANDSTAND / ADHO MUKHA VRKSASANA

In addition to turning the world upside down and being great fun at parties, inversions reverse the flow of blood and lymph. They are thus beneficial for the heart and kidneys. In some traditions, handstand is considered the primary inversion because its actions are less complex than those of the more classically revered head and shoulder stands. All inversions require a leap of faith while cultivating an appreciation for alternative perspectives. Handstand is perhaps the most empowering because it requires a measure of upper body strength and an openness in the shoulder girdle--where many of us are chronically tight.

Benefits: strengthens the arms, wrists, neck and shoulders; conquers fear

Preparation for: handstand without the wall

Contraindications: shoulder and wrist injuries, high blood pressure, heart disease.

Drishti: between the hands.

Do:

- keep forearms squeezing towards each other
- lift the legs and pelvis up from the lower abdomen
- keep the neck released

Pointers:

- shoulder blades draw into spine
- upper arm bones externally rotate
- fingers spread wide
- weight evenly distributed; breath even
- hands stay close to wall so the lower back does not overarch

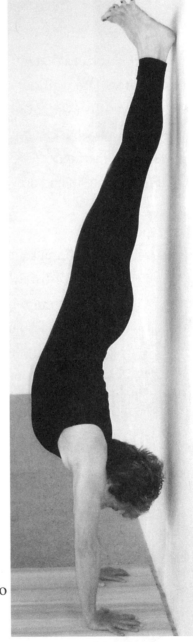

<u>Assist</u>

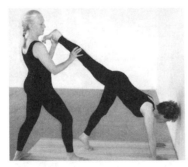 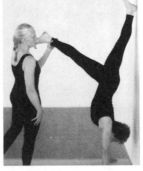

Begin in down dog; press raised ankle into partner's hand to lift; bring hips over shoulders before raising legs.

82

<u>"L" Handstand</u> is identical in shape to Dandasana and Wall Dog, both of which can be used as preparatory asanas. This pose is more challenging for the shoulders than the previous handstand, but it's often more accessible because of the wall's support.

Pointers:

- heels press into wall
- lower abdomen draws in
- shoulder blades on back
- heart moves toward wall
- feet in line with hips
- forearms squeeze in

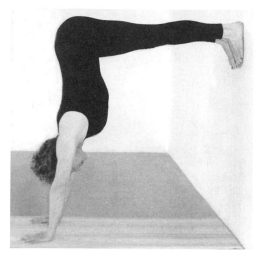

<u>Wall Splits Lift</u>

In this version, the lower foot presses into the wall. This pose mimics warrior III in shape and can be used in preparation for it.

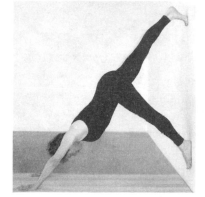

<u>Measuring</u>

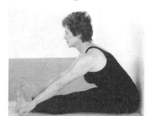

Mark placement of heels; take down dog with heels of hands at that spot; place toes of 1 foot at wall 2-3 inches above sitz bones; press back and lift.

CHAIR / UTKATASANA

This pose gets its English name because of the directive: "Imagine sitting back into a chair." In Sanskrit, it's called "Fierce," which is a bit more apt in terms of the energy required to hold the posture for very long. With the assistance of the wall, however, unseasoned legs are able to remain in the asana with relative ease. Eventually, the spine and legs become supple and strong and fierce pose becomes a friend. The upper arm bones move behind the ears as they externally rotate to assist the lift in the rib cage. This upward action is balanced by the downward movement of the pelvis and a slight tuck in the tailbone.

Benefits: strengthens ankles, thighs, arms and lower back; opens shoulders; stretches ribs and chest; tones abdominal organs and spine

Preparation: for same pose without the wall

Contraindications: sacral and knee issues

Drishti: up, between hands

Do:

- press inner heels and balls of big toes down
- anchor sitz bones and tuck tailbone
- lift lower abdomen

Pointers:

- feet hip distance apart; ankles and knees press toward each other
- shoulder blades draw toward each other and down

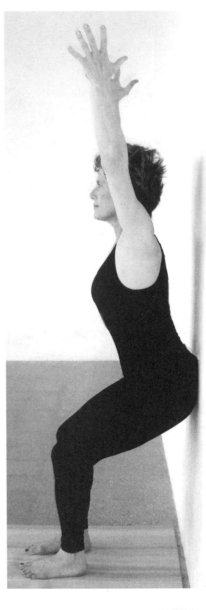

Back at Wall

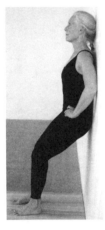

Tuck pelvis, bring shoulder blades back and down. Find comfortable position for lower back. (For sciatic issues, keep lumbar curve.) Once the legs are trained, the torso can move forward into the full pose.

Quad Challenge

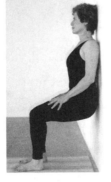

Shoulders and back of head press lightly into wall to take some of the weight off the legs and feet. Quads engage and navel draws in.

Cactus and Eagle Arms

Can be combined to create a dynamic pose by inhaling when the arms expand and exhaling when they close.

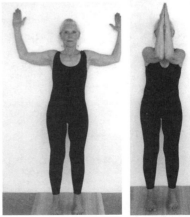

84

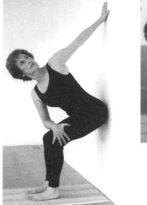
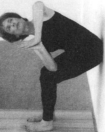

Twists

In both versions the sitz bones press into the wall, the feet are parallel, the hips remain squared and the twisting is done from the navel. The neck extends from the spine: it and the head turn last.

SQUAT / MALASANA

One of the things that's gone by the wayside in developed nations is the ability to squat. People who live in cultures less dependent on indoor plumbing and furniture also have fewer lower back and hip problems than those of us who enjoy the comforts of modern life.

Benefits: releases the lower back and hips; strengthens the ankles; stretches the Achilles tendons; tones the abdomen

Preparation for: squat without the wall

Contraindications: knee pain

Drishti: horizon or tip of nose

Do:

- press inner heels and big toes into floor
- engage quads

Pointers:

- lower abdomen draws in and ribs telescope up
- shoulder blades and back of head press wall

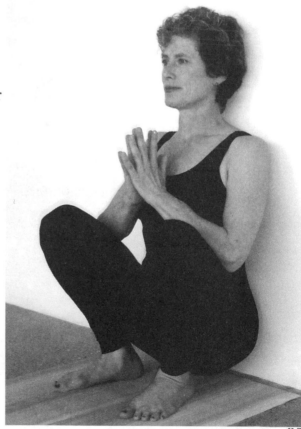

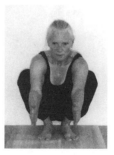

Hugging In

Thighs squeeze arms. Sitz bones press back and down. Shoulder blades draw back as arms reach forward; lower back rounds.

CHILD'S POSE / BALASANA

Known as "wisdom pose" in some traditions, child's pose is the quintessential inward-looking asana.   Both versions offered here are more actively engaging than the customary posture, which utilizes gravity far more than muscular effort.

Benefits:

Opens hips; stretches spine, arms, and neck; releases tension in feet

Preparation for: downward facing dog

Contraindications: knee injuries, low back and hip pain

Drishti: tip of nose, floor

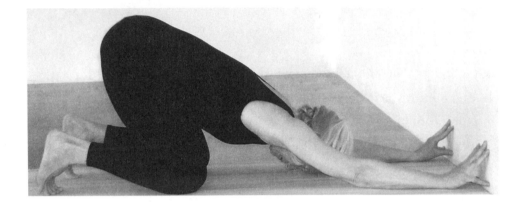

Do:

- press hands into wall
- keep shoulder blades moving toward each other

Pointers:

- sitz bones press towards heels
- lower abdomen draws toward spine
- breath is felt in back of torso

Feet at the Wall
Press balls of feet into wall. Keep knees hip distance apart. Press heels back as if to touch the wall. Reach forward with hands.

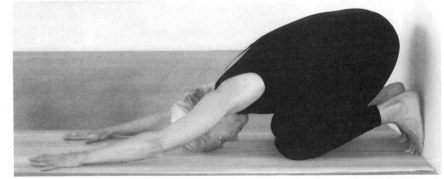

86

TABLE

Table is a foundational pose in that it creates a template for the hands, arms and shoulders that can be applied in down dog in plank and 4-limbed staff pose and in many of the arm balances. Done with the feet at the wall, it encourages active participation of the legs. Done away from the wall, it positions the body for balancing with one foot lifted and pressing into the wall.

Benefits: strengthens arms and wrists; stretches fascia of feet; helps maintain mobility in the toes

Preparation for: downward facing dog, leg extensions

Contraindications: carpal tunnel syndrome, wrist pain

Drishti: between the hands

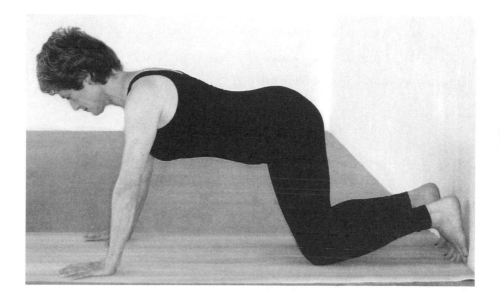

Do:

- spread fingers and distribute weight evenly across the hands
- spread sitz bones
- press on toe pads and balls of feet

Pointers:

- lower abdomen draws towards spine
- knees an inch or two behind hips and hands an inch in front of shoulders
- shoulder blades draw towards each other, lower back ribs near kidneys inflate, upper abdomen softens and lower back arches slightly
- elbows straight but not locked; "eyes" of elbows face thumbs

BRIDGE / SETU BANDHASANA

Also known as dvi pada pitham, two footed lift pose, this version of bridge is both a variation of a more strenuous neck strengthener and an essential pose in a beginner's repertoire. It's the only posture in this book that uses the wall as a point of reference rather then for resistance or support. Alignment is assisted by reaching the knees and shins toward the wall rather than actually pressing into it.

Benefits: strengthens neck, thighs, back and ankles; releases psoas; opens shoulder girdle; stretches groins, chest and ribs

Preparation for: shoulder stand, full bridge, upward facing bow, abdominal work

Contraindications: slipped and/or compressed cervical disks, low back and knee pain

Drishti: tip of nose, up

Do:

- press on balls of feet and inner heels
- direct knees and shins towards wall
- keep throat open and back of neck curved and off the floor

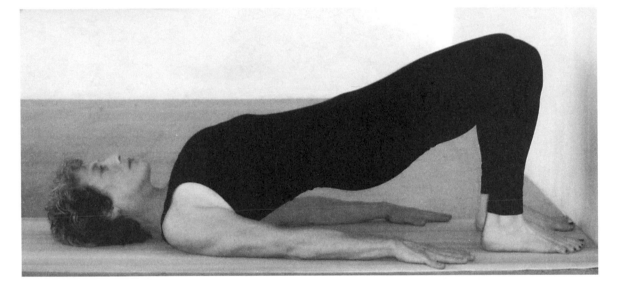

Pointers:

- shins and knees move simultaneously towards wall and towards each other
- arms and hands press into floor
- shoulder blades move towards each other
- back of head presses lightly into floor
- sternum moves towards chin (not sternum towards chin)
- ribs expand as pelvis lifts
- lower abdomen is slightly contracted

Bridge with Block

Press against block to increase engagement of legs. Block can be between knees or close to the pubic bone. Each has a slightly different effect, so experiment.

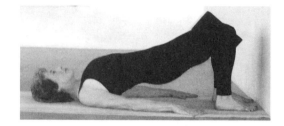

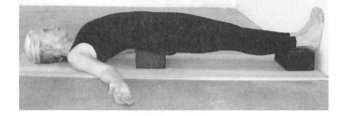

Supported Bridge

A restorative variation that opens both the spine and the heart.

SHOULDER STAND / SALAMBA SARVANGASANA

Called the queen of asanas because of its physiological benefits, shoulder stand requires openness in the shoulder girdle as well as suppleness and strength in the cervical spine. For many of us, this pose is difficult because of the chronic tension we carry in our necks and in the V-shaped trapezius muscles that descend from the shoulders to the spine at heart level. In addition, the lower body must lift up, which requires considerable abdominal strength and control. For these reasons, and becasue of the inherent fagility of the neck, many of us who teach would not consider including this pose in a beginning class. The wall is helpful, however, in assisting the lift and in positioning the pelvis over the shoulders. It makes the posture accessible to many who would otherwise be unable to lift their lower bodies. Shoulder stand is an important asana and one well worth working toward. In fact, its benefits are so numerous that Mr. Iyengar devotes an entire page of *Light on Yoga* to them. A few are listed here.

Benefits: strengthens the neck, arms, hands and shoulders; releases tension in the neck and shoulders; rests the heart; facilitates lymph drainage; regulates the thyroid and parathyroid; relieves constipation; alleviates headaches and sinus congestion; restores vitality; calms the nerves

Preparation for: shoulder stand without the wall

Contraindications: high blood pressure, heart disease, neck injuries, wrist, elbow, shoulder pain

Drishti: tip of nose, up.

(photo on next page)

Do:

- press heels into wall
- keep throat open and natural curve in neck
- keep shoulder blades and elbows drawing towards each other
- slightly contract abdomen and internally rotate thighs

Pointers:

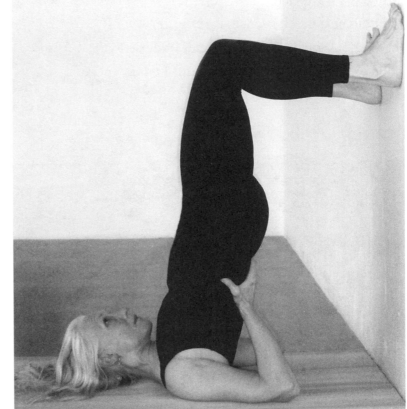

- heels of hands support spine at region of kidneys
- upper arm bones press into floor
- back of head presses lightly into floor as chin moves away from sternum
- torso lifts; ribs telescope towards ceiling
- pubic bone moves towards front plane to align pelvis over shoulders

Supported Sacrum

Less strenuous for the shoulders and neck and accessible to many with cervical disk anomolies.

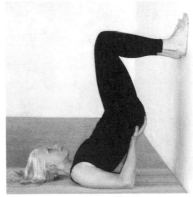

Supported Lumbar Spine
Lower back arched; an intermediate pose that strengthens the lower back.

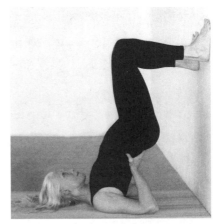

PLOUGH / HALASANA

As the blade of the plough touches the earth, so too do the toe pads press into the floor. Plough is part of the shoulder stand cycle, meaning that it is done in sequence with shoulder stand. As a preparatory pose, it readies the neck to bear the body's weight. As a counterpose, it stretches the postural muscles that can become fatigued while holding the trunk and legs erect over the shoulders.

Benefits: stimulates abdominal organs; stretches spine, shoulders, neck and legs; alleviates flatulence; reduces blood pressure

Preparation for: plough without the wall; shoulder stand

Contraindications: neck injuries and cervical disk problems, heart disease

Drishti: knees, tip of nose

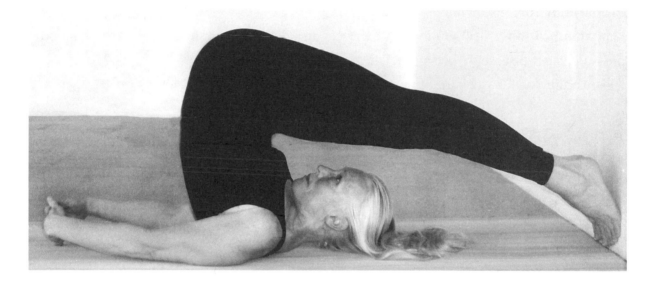

Do:
- press balls of the toes into wall
- maintain slight contraction in lower abdominal muscles
- press lightly on back of head
- keep throat open and back of neck off of the floor

Pointers:
- hamstrings stretch
- legs and hips lift; inner thighs rotate internally
- elbows draw towards each other
- shoulder blades integrate with spine

<u>Legs Parallel with Floor</u>
Heels press into wall; lower belly engaged; neck free; torso and hips lift. The emphasis here is on stretching the spine, neck and shoulders.

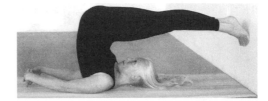

FISH / MATSYASANA

Also part of the shoulder stand cycle, fish is a counterpose for shoulder stand and plough as it alleviates some of the stress that may be experienced in postural muscles unused to holding the pelvis erect or stretching as intensely as halasana encourages.

Benefits: fully expands ribs and chest to increase lung capacity; strengthens lower back and neck; activates thyroid

Preparation for: fish without the wall

Contraindications: neck injuries and cervical disk dislocations, shoulder pain, high blood pressure, heart disease, hyperthyroidism

Drishti: third eye, baseboard of opposite wall

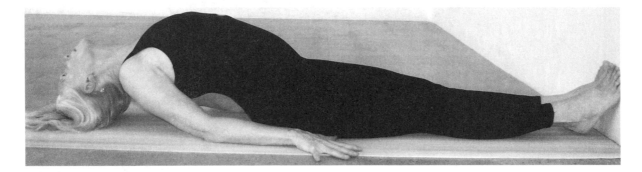

Do:
- press forearms into floor
- press balls of feet into wall
- lift sternum away from navel

Pointers:
- top of pelvis tilts forward
- shoulder blades move towards each other
- elbows remain midway between hips and shoulders
- top of head presses lightly into earth
- throat is open and back of neck is free of compression
- inner thighs rotate down

SPINAL TWIST / JATARA PARIVARTANASANA

Although twisting can be done from a variety of positions, the poses included here endeavor to maintain pelvic stability while rotating the torso on its axis against the resistance of "squared" hips. Note that it's not always possible to maintain the perfect stacking of one hip on the other or the tracking of both hips in the same plane. So think directionally. Squaring the pelvis is the action toward which we aim, resisting the tendency to become skewed by anchoring toward stability. This is especially important for those whose SI joint is unstable since twisting sometimes easily dislocates this joint.

Benefits: tones the abdominal muscles and organs; stimulates kidneys and adrenals; stretches ribs and lower back

Preparation for: same pose without the wall

Contraindications: disc injuries, hiatal hernia

Drishti: to the opposite side

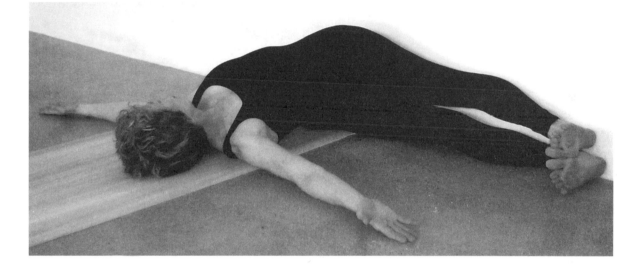

Do:

- press heels into wall
- keep lower abdomen slightly drawn in
- twist from waist

Pointers:

- thighs active
- hips and same side shoulder anchor body
- opposite shoulder moves towards floor
- ribs telescope towards head
- sitz bones at wall

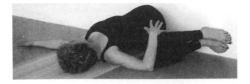

<u>Knees Bent</u>

Top foot presses into the wall to deepen the actions; hand presses thigh to increase leverage.

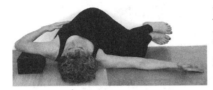

<u>Upper Arm on Block</u>

If the shoulder doesn't reach floor, a block gives support and resistance. Upper arm presses down to increase the effect.

<u>Knees at 90°</u>

Same actions as above but knees retain a 90° bend. Less taxing for the sacrum. Block between knees adds stability.

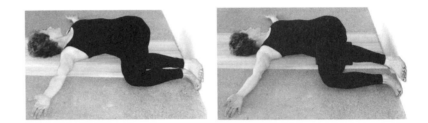

Symmetry: Wide-legged Poses

WIDE LEGGED STANDING FORWARD BEND / PRASARITA PADOTTANASANA

In general, wide-legged forward bends are easier than those in which the legs are close or next to each other. For this reason, they're an important part of any beginning yoga practice. Prasarita means expanded or spread out. Pada refers to the foot. In this pose the spreading of the feet affords an intense stretch to the inner thighs. Without the wall, the head works towards the space between the legs. At the wall the legs are fixed and unable to compensate for the forward movement of the body's weight. Thus, moving the head between the legs is courting a fall. Nonetheless, prasarita at the wall teaches us how to engage the quads and adductors in order to deepen the stretch in the hamstrings. The use of blocks is advised until the muscles let go sufficiently for the pelvis and torso to fold over the heads of the femur bones with comfort.

Benefits: stretches the adductors (inner thighs), the groins, the hamstrings and the muscles along the spine; strengthens the ankles and arches; tones the abdominal organs and the quadriceps; improves digestion and elimination

Preparation for: same pose without the wall; closed-legged forward bends

Contraindications: slippery SI joint

Drishti: tip of nose, floor

Do:

- press heels and sitz bones into wall; hug adductors towards each other
- engage quads and internally rotate inner thighs towards wall
- keep weight evenly distributed on feet--front to back and side to side

Pointers:

- lower abdomen tones
- shoulder blades on back; elbows bend to sides and hands form teepee; neack and head are free
- spine straight; pelvis rotates over heads of femur bones and downward pull of gravity is countered equally by in and upward effort in legs
- sitz bones widen and tailbone lightly tucks

Hands on Blocks

If hands don't reach floor, place hands on blocks underneath shoulders. Keep your ears in line with your shoulders. The crown of your head moves forward.

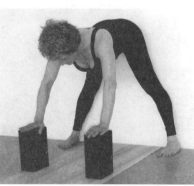

Spinal Twist

Sitz bones press into wall to anchor pelvis; shoulders stack; arms form straightl line; twist from abdomen; turn head last.

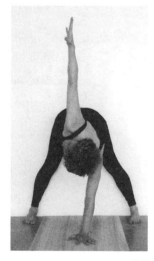

BUTTERFLY, BOUND ANGLE / BADDHA KONASANA

This pose gets its English name from the shape of the legs, which look like the wings of a butterfly. Like butterflies hovering over a flower, beginning students tend to move their legs up and down. The effects of the pose, however, can best be felt by holding the limbs still. The literal translation of the Sanskrit name is "bound angle," which more aptly describes the actions of the feet and legs as they work isometrically, one side in resisting the other to activate the quadriceps of both. This isometric effort--equal and opposite--begins to bring the knees closer to the floor. Working with the wall creates spinal stability, helps to maintain the lumbar curve, and allows some of us to settle more fully into the sensations in our hips.

Benefits: stretches groins, inner thighs, and hips; strengthens pelvic floor and ankles; brings blood into pelvis, abdomen, and lower back; alleviates menstrual difficulties and sciatic pain

Preparation for: same pose without the wall

Contraindications: knee and hip pain

Drishti: tip of nose or horizon

Do:

- press feet together
- bring heels near perineum
- draw lower abdomen in

Pointers:

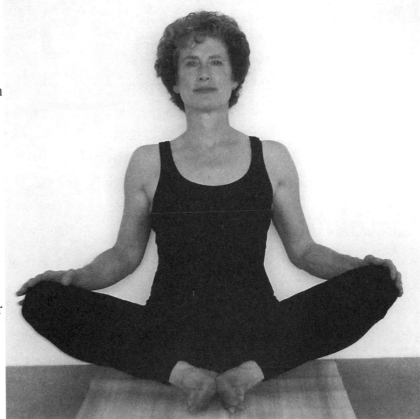

- inner thighs and quadriceps engage
- knees work towards floor
- spine erect with lumbar curve in place
- shoulder blades move towards or press into wall
- back of head lightly presses wall

96

EASY POSE / SIDDHASANA

This asana's English name belies its importance. It's true that it's an easier seat for meditation than lotus, but the extraordinary states of mind attained through meditation are available even in this simple asana. Thus the Sanskrit "Siddhasana" reflects the posture's potential to become a vehicle for attaining higher levels of consciousness and bliss. A siddha is a semi-Divine being; the siddhis are supernatural powers. Siddhasana, therefore, is not just *easy;* it's also essential to yoga, the merging of self with Self.

Benefits: relaxes the entire body, calms the mind; helps maintain flexibility in hips, knees, and ankles.

Preparation for: easy pose without the wall, meditation, pranayama (breathing exercises)

Contraindications: ankle, knee, hip injuries

Drishti: tip of nose, horizon

Do:

- maintain slight contraction in lower abdomen
- maintain curve in lower back
- externally rotate inner thighs

Pointers:

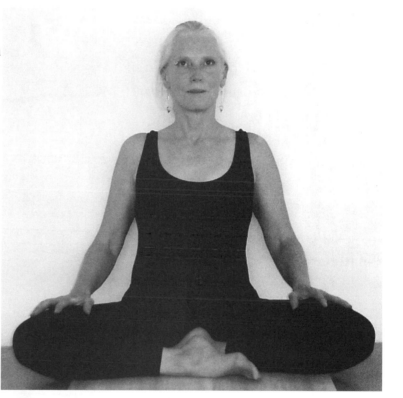

- shoulder blades draw towards each other
- ribs telescope up
- pelvis grounds
- torso lifts out of pelvis base
- back of head presses back

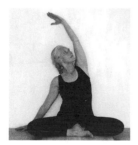

Side Bend

Anchor sitz bones; lift, then bend; stretch one side without compressing the other.

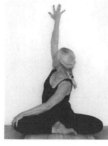

Twist

Press one hand against thigh and othe into wall; twist from navel.

Asymmetry: Closed-hipped Poses

WARRIOR I / VIRABHADRASANA I

      This posture is named after the legendary hero, Virabhadra, who is said to have arisen from a discarded hair that Shiva threw down in anger over the death of his wife, Sati. Virabhadra avenged Shiva's loss and is ever immortalized with this and two other poses that bear his name. Because of the twist that occurs in the back leg, this warrior is one of the most complex of the standing poses and one of the ones that benefit most from using the wall.

Benefits: stretches and strengthens legs, hips and ankles; expands chest; relieves tension in the neck and shoulders; tones lower back expands chest, cultivates balance

Preparation for: warrior I without the wall and warrior III

Contraindications: neck, knee, hip and lower back pain, high blood pressure

Drishti: between hands or the horizon

Do:

- press the back heel into the wall
- press the ball and inner heel of the forward foot down
- slightly tuck tailbone
- maintain slight contraction of lower abdominal muscles
- keep forward knee over or slightly behind ankle

Pointers:

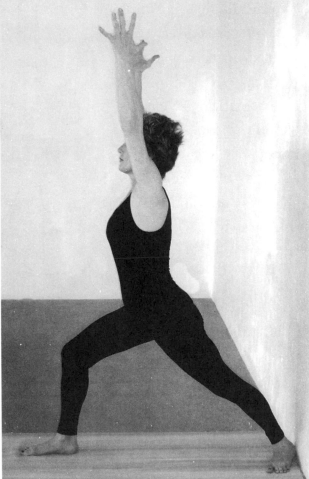

- back hip moves forward and back thigh rotates internally; toes turn in
- upper arms move behind ears; head moves back
- knee remains in same plane as hip and ankle
- back calf twists slightly
- front thigh externally rotates
- torso lifts out of pelvis and shoulder blades move towards each other

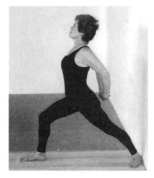

Hands Interlaced behind Back

This variation opens the chest and increases space in the thoracic cavity. It releases tension in the shoulders and shoulder blades. The same actions in the feet, legs, pelvis and torso apply as when the arms are raised. *Note: the elbows are slightly bent as they draw up; hands interlace; neck is open and shoulder blades move down spine.*

CRESCENT WARRIOR / VIRABHADRASANA I VARIATION

Although balance is a little more challenging in this pose than it is with the back heel on the floor, it's less complex than the previous asana. This is due to the fact that the back heel is off the ground, which maintains a tidy alignment between the ankle, knee, and hip. It also facilitates greater mobility and control of the back foot for beginning students. Once the legs become stable, the torso can assume numerous shapes, many of which reflect those of other standing poses for a similar effect.

Benefits: strengthens thighs, calves, ankles, feet, and lower back; opens shoulders, psoas, and groins; expands chest, cultivates balance

Preparation for: same pose without the wall, warrior I

Contraindications: neck injuries (don't look up), high blood pressure, low back and knee pain

Drishti: between hands or the horizon

Do:

- tack the back heel to the wall
- press the ball of the front big toe down
- lift torso out of pelvis
- maintain slight contraction of lower abdominal muscles
- keep forward knee over or slightly behind ankle

Pointers:

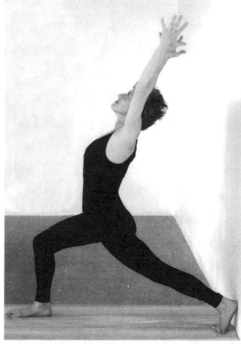

- shoulder blades draw in and down
- upper arms externally rotate
- sitz bones widen
- front thigh externally rotates
- back thigh lifts and spins inward

99

<u>Vertical Spine</u>
Decreases lumbar arch to improve comfort. Look at the horizon and keep wrists, elbows, shoulders, and hips in the same vertical plane.

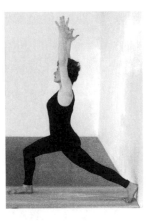

LUNGE / ANAJANI ASANA

Anajani, a monkey girl, is said to have been ravaged by Lord Vayu, god of the wind. Hanuman was the progeny of this union between a lowly animal and the Divine. From the moment of his birth, Hanuman was devoted to Rama, an incarnation of Vishnu, the vital essence that lives within and preserves all life. A white monkey with a playful attitude, Hanuman was adept at many things. One of these was his ability to leap great distances. In order to find and save Rama's wife Sita from the clutches of Ravana, king of the demons, Hanuman jumped across the southern sea from the tipi of India to Sri Lanka. To commemorate this event, splits pose, hanumanasana, is named after him.

Before we can attempt such an extreme stretch, our hamstrings, psoas and groins must be open. Thus the lunge is named for Hanuman's mother. Anjani asana prepares the legs for the pose that commemorates her son. It's an important conditioning asana in its own right, however, since our sedentary lives tend to bind not only our groins, but also the psoas, which lunging also releases. There are marked similarities between the lunge and crescent warrior, most notably in the hip flexor muscles and in the lower back. The primary difference is one of balance, which is easier with the one knee on the floor. In either pose, once the legs and hips are stable and secure, the torso may twist, arch and bend to vary the overall effects.

Note that when the back knee is on the floor, bringing the forward knee beyond the foot is both safe and helpful for stretching the psoas and groins as long as the inner front heel is kept down. In their various forms, both crescent warrior and anjani asana address a chronically shortened psoas and are, therefore, some of the most important preparatory poses for all of the standing asanas.

Benefits: stretches groins, calves, arches, ankles, thighs and psoas; strengthens quadriceps; tones abdomen

Preparation for: lunging without the wall, splits, warrior I & II, crescent warrior

Contraindications: groin injuries, low back pain

Drishti: 3rd eye, hands, place where ceiling meets wall

Do:

- press back heel into wall
- move forward knee and shin towards center of room
- maintain even weight distribution on both feet
- llightly tuck tailbone

Pointers:

- thigh bones draw into pelvis to square hips
- back thigh lifts and rotates internally
- sitz bones widen
- sternum moves away from navel
- chest lifts; ribs telescope up; upper arms externally rotate
- lower abdomen draws in

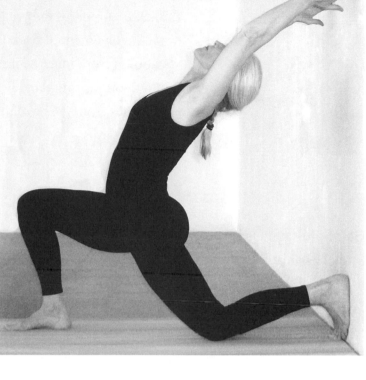

Hands on Blocks
Enables torso to lift off of leg so that hips, legs, ankles and feet can align.

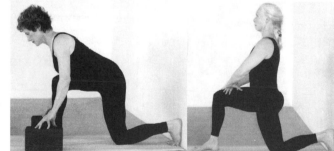

Hands on Knee
Hands press against thigh, shoulder blades draw towards each other.

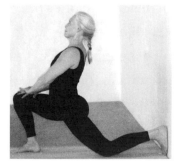

Psoas & Groin Openers
In both, forward knee moves beyond the ankle and corresponding hip moves back. Back foot presses into wall as its hip comes forward.

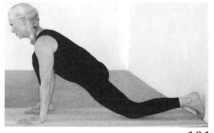

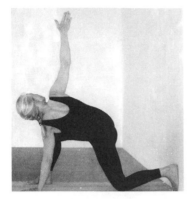

Closed Twists

Back foot presses into wallfor active involvement of back leg and stability; front inner heel presses into floor; hips remain level; twist emanates from the navel; balanced effort in arms.

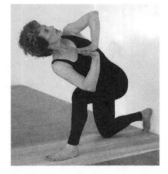

Half Splits and Quad Stretches are not part of the Anjani family; nonetheless, they're presented here because follow intuitively from the lunges.

Half Splits

Front heel anchors as the ball of the big toe points forward and the toe pads flex back; thigh bone draws back; hips move towards square.

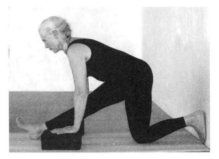

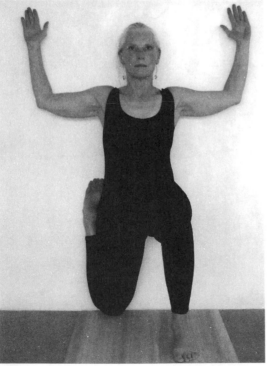

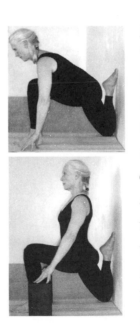

Quad Stretches:

Toes of back foot fan against wall; shin and foot press into wall as sitz bone and thigh move toward wall; eventually, heels nests along inner edge of back foot; ball of front big toe and inner heel press into floor and forward knee aligns with hip and ankle.

PIGEON / EKA PADA RAJAKAPOTASANA

This pose follows nicely from the lunge in that it builds on the groin opening of the previous posture. Openness as well as a measure of communication with the hip and back leg are both necessary in order to stabilize the pelvis as the forward thigh rotates externally. Although most commonly thought of as a pose for the hips, once these become supple enough that the pelvis is secure, the torso lifts out of the lower body to expand the chest. The body then resembles a pigeon with its chest puffed. Hence the Sanskrit name: One Legged King Pigeon Pose. In most beginning classes pigeon is taught with the torso folded over the bent forward leg, which places leverage deep inside the hip to stretch the tissues.

Benefits: stretches feet, legs, groins, psoas and hips; aligns sacrum; strengthens ankles and knees; alleviates sciatic pain

Preparation for: king pigeon pose with erect spine and without the wall

Contraindications: knee injuries

Drishti: tip of nose

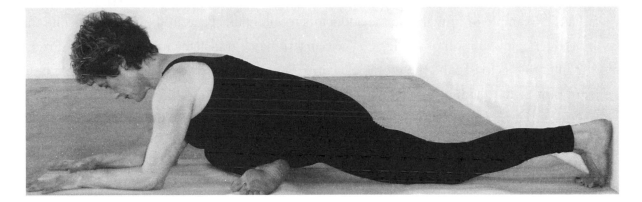

Do:
- keep back heel pressing into wall
- maintain even weight distribution on both legs
- engage lower abdomen

Pointers:
- back hip widens as back thigh rotates internally
- gluteals relaxed
- thighs hug to midline
- front foot flexed with active toes; outer edge presses into floor
- front knee wider than front hip
- tail bone tucks

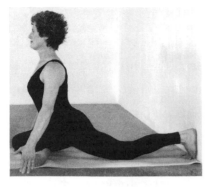

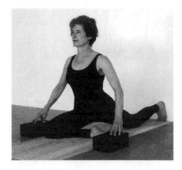

<u>Spine Erect</u>

Strengthens the lower back and expands the chest wall. Anchor legs and hips; lift torso out of pelvis; maintain tuck in tailbone; square hips; draw shoulder blades towards each other. Back foot, ankle, knee and hip align. Can place hands on blocks to assist lift.

RUNNER'S STRETCH / PARSVOTTANASANA II

Because of the positioning of the feet, legs and hips, this pose is part of the warrior I family of poses, which include that warrior and revolved triangle. While the hips never completely square up, they move in that direction, getting resistance from the feet, which anchor the pose and help to stretch the legs. Because the inner thighs are active in this pose, it's a classic example of how to use the adductors to maintain space in the sacrum despite the asymmetrical configuration of the legs. The Sanskrit name translates as "Side Stretch Pose," and the intention is to expand the thoracic cavity. This is, however, not entirely possible until we learn how to use the hips and legs to create a base from which to lengthen the torso. Here we're concentrating on the hamstrings and legs, which need to become both elastic and strong before the chest can expand.

Benefits: stretches hamstrings, calves, ankles, spine; strengthens ankles; tones abdominals

Preparation for: same pose without the wall, warrior I, revolved triangle

Contraindications: high blood pressure (keep spine parallel to floor), heart disease

Drishti: 2nd toe on forward foot, knee

(photo on next page)

Do:

- bring forward hip back and back hip forward
- use adductors to decompress sacrum and align spine and pelvis
- draw lower abdomen in

Pointers
- outer edge of back heel presses into wall
- ball of forward big toe presses lightly into floor
- quads of forward leg lift
- back lengthens
- weight evenly distributed on both feet

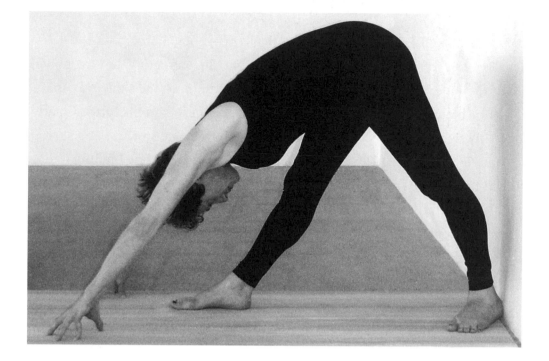

Hands on Blocks

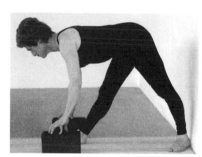

Spine parallel with floor, hands press with equal effort into blocks to assist stretch of spine.

Fingers Interlaced

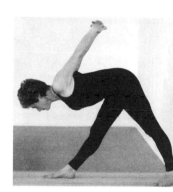

The arms assist the stretching of the thoracic cavity to increase lung space and capacity.

Funky Foot

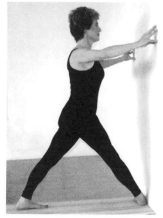

Outer edge of front foot presses into and outer edge of front shin moves toward wall; forward hip draws back as back hip draws forward. Inner back heel presses down as both thighs internally rotate. Tailbone slightly tucks. Used as a transitional pose in a flow, this posture stretches the ankles, calves, legs and hips in some unique ways.

REVOLVED TRIANGLE / PARIVRITTA TRIKONASANA

This relative of warrior I is especially useful for correcting hip anomalies since it makes use of the inner thighs to decompress the sacrum in much the same way that squeezing a blanket roll or block between the knees brings the tops of the thighs farther apart, which in turn pulls gently against the pelvis from inside the hip to create space at the sacroiliac joint. Revolved triangle is also one of the most difficult poses in the warrior I family to do. Balance is crucial, and this comes from working the hips toward square as well as from maintaining a steady back leg. Revolving around the axis of the spine, the torso finds equilibrium through its three points of contact (feet and 1 hand) with the eath.

Benefits: strengthens legs, ankles and lower back; stretches the ribs and chest, creating optimal space for the lungs and breathing; opens the hips and massages internal organs.

Preparation for: same pose without the wall

Contraindications: low back pain

Drishti: to the side and up

Do:

- press back heel into wall
- square hips
- engage inner thighs

Pointers:

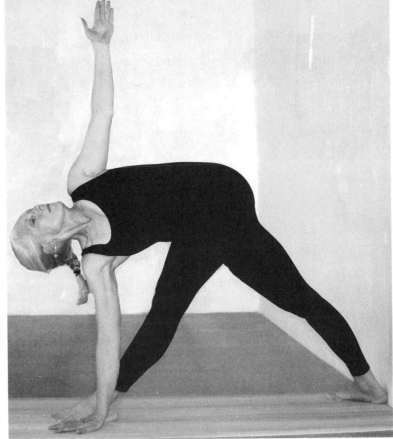

- forward hip draws back; back hip draws forward
- spine parallel with floor; sides lengthen
- twist from waist
- shoulder blades in
- arms form straight line
- head turns last

106

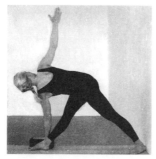

<u>With Block</u>
If hamstrings are inelastic, use a block, or place the hand on the floor on the inside of your foot. You can also press lightly on your shin. If the upper shoulder is tight, place that hand on your waist.

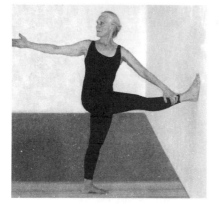

<u>Foot on Wall</u>
This relative of extended hand-to-foot pose is placed here because its shape is similar to that of revolved triangle. The hips remain level, the quads engage and the standing foot turns out slightly. The forward hand and raised leg work isometrically against each other.

<u>Supine Spinal Twists</u>
Both of these poses teach the shape of revolved triangle. The straight leg is engaged as the foot presses the wall; hips stack and anchor; twist emanates from navel.

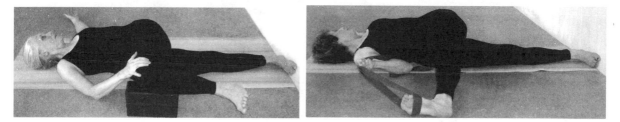

WARRIOR III / VIRABHADRASANA III

One of my favorites to teach at the wall, this pose benefits greatly from a partner assist. It requires abdominal control and an understanding of the role the raised back leg plays in maintaining balance. It can also be considered the next step in the sequence from Parsvottanasana. The angle between the legs is slightly larger, but the actions established in the Runner's Stretch are similar. In addition, the pelvic stability attained in the previous pose is helpful in establishing and maintaining spinal equilibrium with the trunk and arms moving in the opposite direction of the back leg and heel. Of all the standing poses, this one most assuredly demonstrates the pivotal role of the core.

Benefits: strengthens the spine, abdomen and legs; tones the arms and neck; cultivates grace, balance. one-pointedness and spinal alignment

Preparation for: warrior III without the wall

Contraindications: low back pain, sciatica

Drishti: third eye, tip of nose, floor

Do:

- press raised foot into wall
- draw lower abdomen in
- reach forward from the navel

Pointers:

- hips work towards being level
- inner thighs activated
- equal and opposite effort/lines of energy from pelvis to wall and from pelvis to center of room
- hip of standing leg anchors pelvis and spine, which is parallel to floor
- spine integrates to level the shoulders; crown of head moves forwa

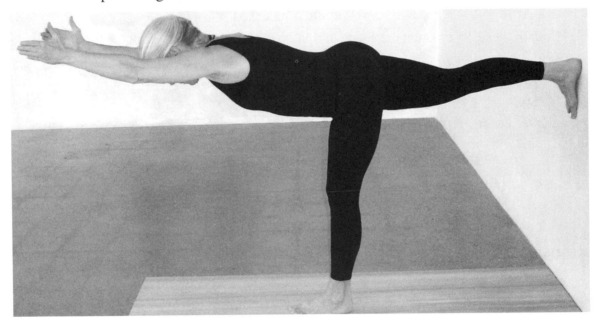

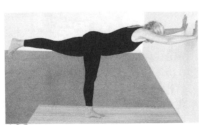

Hands at Wall
Hands press wall;
toes flex toward
knee.

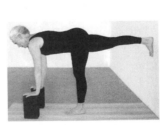

Hands on Blocks
Blocks under
shoulders; hips
level.

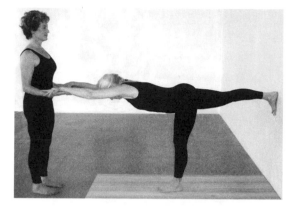

Partner Assist

Partner Assist

Partner not only assists balance but also coaches hip and shoulder alignment and offers something tangible to reach for with the hands. *Assistants, be mindful of your posture. Keep your spine erect and your elbows close to your ribs. Place palms up; do not pull your partner's hands forward.*

Sunbird

Not identical in actions but close enough to be useful in learning them. Use abdominals and spinal muscles to keep hips level; shoulder blades integrate with spine and back toes point down.

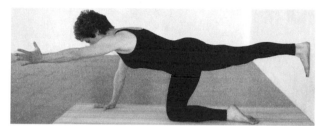

EXTENDED HAND TO BIG TOE POSE / UTTHITA HASTA PADANGUSTHASANA

For many of my students, tight hamstrings restrict forward bending and become the site of extreme resistance within other poses as well. Extended hand to big toe pose stretches these muscles; simultaneously, it develops the quadriceps and opens the groins. It's a lovely pose but requires considerable balance to do well. Using the wall allows us to concentrate on opening and strengthening without worrying about whether or not we're going to fall over. Used wisely, the wall can also cultivate the balance we seek by giving us the freedom to learn to use our muscles to create and maintain equilibrium in the posture. As with warrior III, the core is pivotal. In addition, aligning the pelvis imparts stability to the legs and feet, and also creates an anchor from which to lift the upper body. There's a slight forward movement of the torso as it approaches the thigh.

Benefits: stretches hamstrings; develops balance, focus, and poise; strengthens leg and arm muscles

Preparation for: all one-legged balance poses

Contraindications: rotator cuff and shoulder blade injuries (don't bring blade forward)

Drishti: tip of nose, horizon, big toe

(photo on next page)

Do:

- keep hips level
- draw thigh bone into hip socket as heel presses forward into wall

Pointers:

- lower abdominals draw towards spine
- pelvis tucks
- spine is erect
- torso lifts out of pelvis; then folds towards leg
- inner heel and ball of standing foot press floor as quads engage
- groins remain spacious

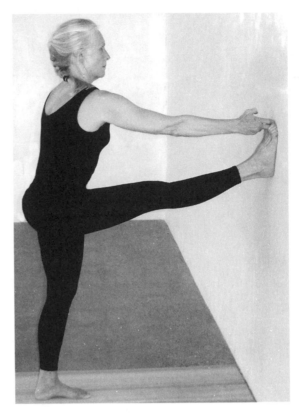

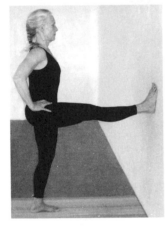

Hands on Hips

Stretches hamstrings; teaches balance. Engage lower abdomen and quads. Press foot into wall; draw thigh bone into hip; bring shoulder blades and elbows towards each other.

Hands and Knee at Wall

Useful for tight hamstrings or lower back pain. Keep hips level and raised leg active by flexing toes and pressing knee into wall. Spine erect, head and neck relaxed quads engaged.

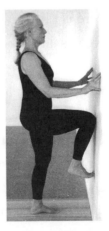

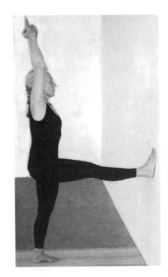

Arms Up

Mimics warrior III and is thus useful for training the body to understand the shape of that posture. Upper arms move behind ears, chin level with horizon, belly drawn in and tailbone tucked. Press into inner heel and lift torso.

110

Back to Wall

These variations give more support than their foot-at-the-wall siblings. Once the standing leg is strong, the raised leg can be conditioned by bringing the hands to the waist to work the quads and core.

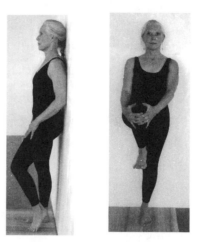

SUPINE HAND TO BIG TOE POSE / SUPTA PADANGUSTHASANA

The beauty of the following series of poses is that balance is taken out of the equation. As a result, students can focus on opening, stretching, and maintaining equilibrium of effort, all of which are important aspects of the standing pose. Thus the supine versions can be considered training grounds as well as templates for utthita hasta padangusthasana. In the reclining version, the abdominals work to lift the torso and the spine rounds slightly, reflecting the shape of its standing cousin.

Benefits: creates awareness of hips, groins, inner heels and thighs; stretches hamstrings; strengthens abdominals

Preparation for: the erect version as well as for many of the standing poses

Contraindications: rotator cuff and shoulder blade injuries (don't bring blade forward)

Drishti: tip of nose, horizon, big toe

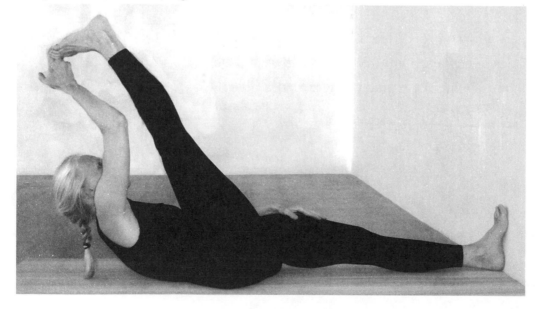

Do:
- press inner heel and ball of big toe into wall
- internally rotate inner thigh of straight leg towards floor

Pointers:
- lower abdominals draw toward spine
- shoulder blades integrate on spine
- thigh bones hug into pelvis
- abdominals lift torso
- neck and shoulders are relaxed
- groins free

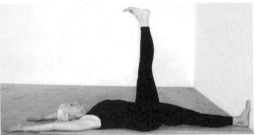

Leg Straight, Arms Back

Encourages lumbar arch; expands the ribs and chest; leg is supported by quads; lower thigh internally rotates as inner edge of foot presses wall to maintain pelvic stability.

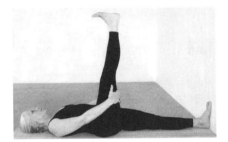

Hands Behind Thigh

Arms and leg engage isometrically to maintain the lumbar arch.

With Strap

Experiment with strap at different places on the foot---heel, balls of toes, arch---each affords slightly different actions. Keep elbows slightly bent and shoulder blades integrated on back.

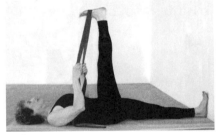

Leg to Side

In both variations, the straight leg resists the movement of the opposite leg by internally rotating the thigh and pressing against the inner heel.

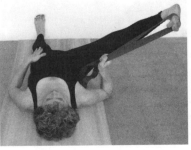
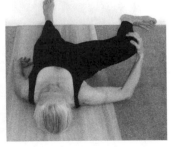

112

Asymmetry: Open-hipped Poses

WARRIOR II / VIRABHADRASANA II

When I hold this pose for very long, I'm reminded that the greatest warfare we can wage takes place within ourselves. Strenuous and deeply engaging, warrior II is challenging on many levels. But when the body becomes comfortable with it, the pose confers an unparalleled sense of vibrancy and strength. In addition, because of the relationship between the legs, this pose becomes a template for the ones that follow in this section; extended side angle, triangle, and half moon all share the open back hip, the abducted and externally rotated front leg and the tucking of the forward hip. Working with the back hand at the wall helps prevent the forward lean that's so common for many of us when we first encounter this posture.

Benefits: strengthens the thighs, calves, and ankles; stretches the groins; tones the abdominal muscles, the abdominal organs, and the arms

Preparation for: warrior II without the wall, extended side angle

Contraindications: knee and hip pain

Drishti: forward hand

Do:

- maintain even weight distribution on both feet
- keep forward knee moving towards outer edge of forward foot
- keep lower abdominals slightly contracted

Pointers:

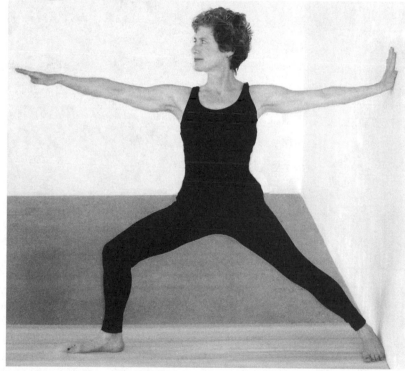

- torso erect
- fingers of back hand press into wall
- shoulder blades on back
- back foot presses into wall

EXTENDED SIDE ANGLE / UTTHITA PARSVAKONASANA

This asana is also known as "Swimmer's Pose" because of the spinal rotation generated by the reach of the forward arm. The relationship of the arm and trunk to the pelvis is similar to that of a person rolling open in the water for a breath during one phase of the crawl stroke.

Benefits: strengthens thighs, calves, ankles; stretches trunk and arms; opens shoulders and hips; encourages digestion and elimination

Preparation for: same pose without the wall

Contraindications: knee and hip pain

Drishti: upstretched hand

Do:

- press forward arm into forward leg and leg into arm
- draw navel and lower abdomen in
- twist from the waist
- keep back leg active

Pointers:

- forward knee tracks in line with hip and ankle
- back thigh finds equilibrium through balanced action of external and internal rotations
- forward thigh externally rotates
- forward hip tucks under
- torso lifts and opens from pelvis

Facing Wall

Fingers press into wall to increase the leverage and spin in the forward arm. Shoulder blades draw towards each other to assist rotation of trunk.

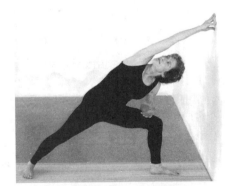

<u>Forearm on Thigh</u>   <u>Hand on Block</u>

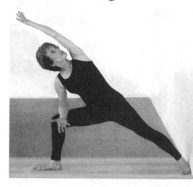 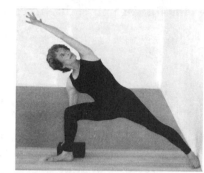

Both of these versions are useful for students whose hands don't reach the floor or if the forward hip begins to bind.

<u>Back at the Wall</u>
Helps students feel shoulder blades; assists understanding of slight backward spin in torso; affords tactile understanding of spiraling the raised arm and the balanced actions of the arm and forward leg. Shoulder blades press wall.

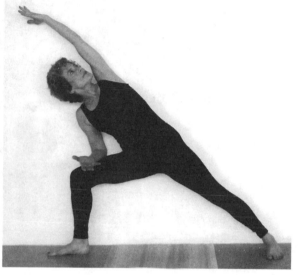

TRIANGLE / UTTHITA TRIKONASANA

Extended triangle is a foundational pose. It's also a pose in which intermediate and advanced students can continually rediscover themselves. Highly nuanced leg and pelvic actions make the unfolding of this posture a continual adventure. One of the foundational actions is the rooting of the ball of the forward big toe.

Benefits: stretches the hamstrings, calves, ankles and arches; strengthens the legs and torso; opens the thoracic cavity and the meridians running through the arms and chest as well as the groins and hips; stabilizes the pelvis

Preparation for: triangle without the wall

Contraindications: neck injuries, sacroiliac and low back pain

Drishti: towards the raised hand

(photo on next page)

115

Do:

- widen (externally rotate) the forward inner thigh; telescope ribs away from pelvis
- draw the thigh bones into the pelvis
- distribute your weight evenly on both feet

Pointers:

- forward hip tucks under
- lower abdomen draws in
- arms form a straight line of energy with each other through the heart
- torso twists slightly back from waist
- ball of forward big toe presses down
- outer edge of back foot presses into wall

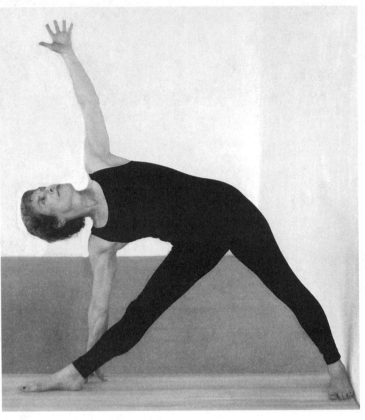

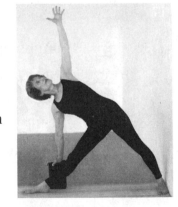

Hand on Block
Useful variation for those with tight hamstrings. Hand can also be placed on thigh, shin, or ankle.

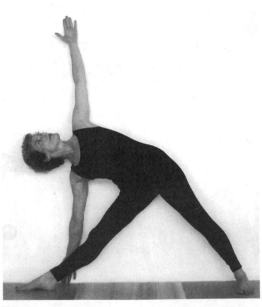

Back at Wall
Outer edge of front foot 3" from wall. Upper shoulder blade presses into wall; forward hip presses into wall; torso leans into wall above actively stable hips and legs. Can be done with a block or with hand on shin or thigh.

HALF MOON / ARDHA CHANDRASANA

This pose can be a challenge for students in that it requires abdominal control as well as a good deal of engagement in the raised leg, which must press back in order to maintain balance against the weight of the torso and arms. The fulcrum is the pelvis, which must be simultaneously stable and spacious. Once mastered, half moon conveys a delicious sense of weightlessness and freedom.

Benefits: strengthens the quads, knees, calves, and ankles; promotes digestion, circulation, and an increase of energy in the back body; opens the hips and chest; improves balance; cultivates an open heart and sense of well being

Preparation for: half moon without the wall

Contraindications: ankle, knee, and neck injuries (don't look up), low blood pressure, vertigo

Drishti: to the side and up

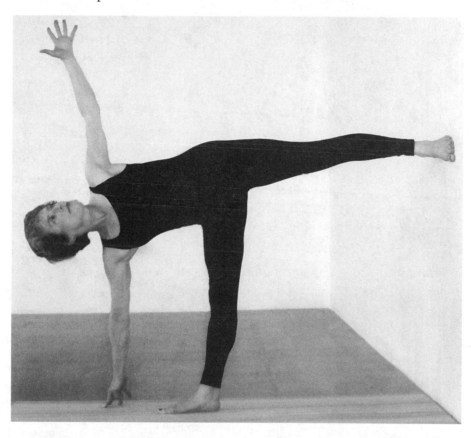

Do:

- maintain core control by slightly contracting the perineum
- engage thighs/quads on both legs; keep ribs telescoping away from hips
- lift the upper hip above the lower and align lower hip over ankle

- keep the back heel in line w/the inner edge of the forward hip
- press foot into wall

Pointers:

- bottom hand underneath lower shoulder; bottom hip under upper one
- head turns towards raised hand; neck is extension of spine
- lower abdomen drawn in
- spine twists slightly (from waist) away from standing leg

<u>With Block</u>
Block assists balance and brings head, neck, torso and leg into straight line, parallel with floor.

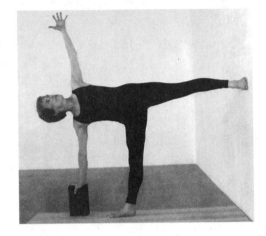

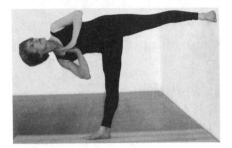

<u>Prayer Hands</u>
Demonstrates importance of back leg.

<u>Back at Wall</u>

This pose is the closest thing to flying I know. There's a delicious weightlessness about it as the body leans into the wall, accepting its support. Upper shoulder and raised heel press into wall.

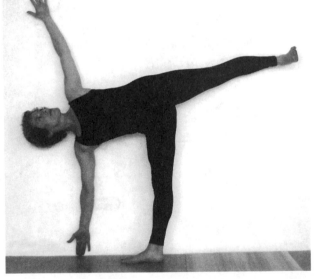

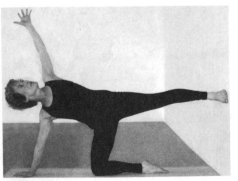

<u>Kneeling</u>
Enjoyable preparatory variation. Engage bottom leg.

118

TREE / VRKSASANA

Tree pose is probably the most stable of the standing balance poses. For this reason, it's considered a foundational pose. Its stability comes from the mutual actions of the legs, which press into one another with equal intensity. Despite its inherent equilibrium, many students find it challenging. The versions depicted below use the wall to bring the challenge away from balance and into strengthening the standing leg and learning work with isometric effort in the legs--foot into leg and leg against foot. A wall is particularly helpful for persons who have bunions or plantar fasciaitis or other foot conditions that make balance difficult. Shown first is my favorite version because it brings the standing hip into alignment with its corresponding knee and ankle.

Benefits: strengthens and tones the ankles, knees, and legs; opens the groins and hips; stretches the spine and torso; fosters concentration and balance; cultivates poise

Preparation for: tree without the wall, all other standing balance poses

Contraindications: ankle, leg and hip pain

Drishti: to the horizon

Do:

- press inner heel and ball of big toe into floor
- press foot into leg and leg into foot
- lift torso up out of pelvis

Pointers:

- bent knee presses lightly into wall
- lower abdomen draws in
- shoulder blades down back and in

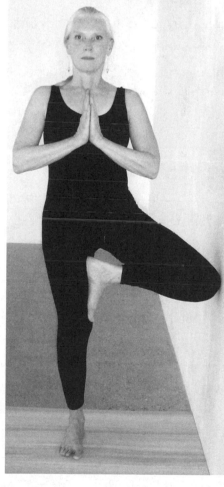

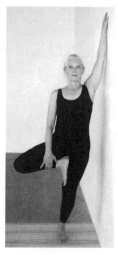

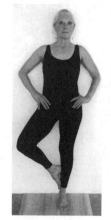

Hand to Wall
Hand maintains light contact with wall; opposite hand at ankle, waist or raise; foot on ankle, calf, thigh or grazing floor.

Back to Wall

Core Cultivation

Both stability and flexibility are necessary in yoga and in life.   In the *Yoga Sutras*, Patanjali calls these qualities *sthira* and *sukha,* firm and yielding. Our pelvic and shoulder girdles need to be firm enough to bear weight evenly and mobile enough to carry us and that which *we* carry with us on our daily rounds.   Linking the girdle at the lower end of the trunk with that at its upper extremity, our core serves to integrate the actions of our limbs and trunk.   Our "core" is commonly thought to refer to our abdominal muscles, particularly the segmented *rectus abdominis* that stretch from just above the pubic bone to just about the middle of the ribs. Typically, core strengtheners involve crunches or leg lifts or a combination of the two. Anything that flexes the trunk and legs towards each other, however, will shorten (and therefore strengthen) the abdominals. If weight bearing is involved, both effort and results are increased.

In addition to the abdominal muscles, the word "core" in yoga also refers to the interior of one's bio-energetic self. What this means is that our core extends the length of our spine and can be experienced through internal movement from the base of the tailbone into the torso and throat and head. The following core cultivating practices sometimes employ movement to get this energy flowing.

BOAT / NAVASANA

In the Ashtanga tradition, boat is the gold standard core cultivator. It utilizes the lower abdominals, the posas, and the pelvic floor to flex the legs and trunk towareds each other--all the while balancing on the sitz bones.   Until the lower belly becomes strong and communication is established between these muscles and the breath, students have difficulty maintaining the deep valley between the legs and torso. The effort of the pose is therefore shifted to the legs, hips, and spine--sometimes with not-so-comfortable results. Using the wall to prop the legs is an intermediate step in gaining control and awareness, as is pressing the heels of the hands against the outer edges of the shins, directly below the knees. Placed thus, the hands fuse the torso and the legs into place without actually supporting either.

Benefits: tones abdomen and quadriceps; alleviates bloating and stimulates elimination; tones kidneys; promotes balance and focus

Preparation for: boat without the wall

Contraindications: lower back and sacral issues (place hands on floor behind hips)

Drishti: toes, tip of nose

(photo on next page)

120

Do:

- draw lower abdomen towards spine and engage pelvic floor
- press heels of hands into outer shins
- bring torso and thighs equally towards each other

Pointers:

- both feet press into and hug wall
- inner ankles and big toes touch; thighs rotate internally; adductors hug in
- sternum lifts away from navel; ribs telescope up; weight balances on sitz bones
- neck relaxed; chin level with horizon
- elbows remain bent and high knees to bring shoulder blades towards each other; to cultivate postural integrity and to eliminate strain on the lower back

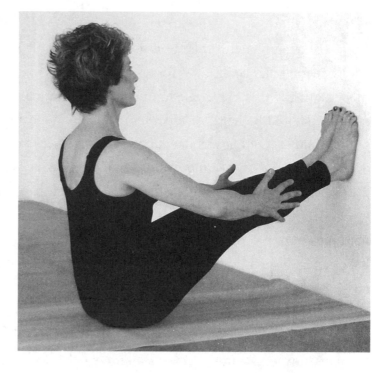

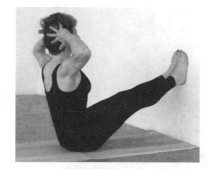

<u>Hands behind Head</u>

Press head into hands; keep shoulder blades on back; maintain posture by pressing into inner heels and lifting the perineum.

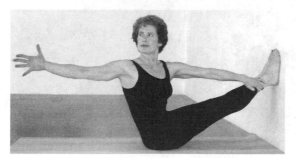

<u>Twisting</u>

Can be held or done with breath-generated movement: exhale into twist and inhale out of it; work dynamically or hold.

TUCKS

The template for this series is the table tuck, in which the 3 points of contact--arms and 1 leg--become the stabilizing forces within the body so that the free leg can move toward the ribs. Not shown is the extension that comes after each tuck. Thus, although the leg flexion may and should be held for a period of time, it's most often followed by a leg lift. Thus the spine rounds and arches as in cat/cow. On the knees or in down dog, there's the added benefit of pressing the foot into the wall when the leg moves back. This opens the groins and frees the psoas. During the first leg extension, pause to align the leg and hips and to feel the pranic opening. Once your body understands the actions, introduce movement into the asana using your inhalations to draw into the body and your exhalations to expand. In all of the tucks, the knee can be brought towards the elbow on the same or opposite side of the body or towards the nose.

Benefits: strengthens abdominals, spine, shoulders, and quadriceps; cultivates awareness of the role the core and shoulders play in stabilizing the body; stretches spine and ankles.

Preparation for: arm balances, sunbird (can be done with sunbird by moving from one to the other--exhale and tuck, inhale and extend foot to wall)

Contraindications: wrist injuries and debilities, carpal tunnel syndrome.

Drishti: tip of nose, navel.

Do:
- engage lower abdomen bring leg forward; i.e. hug in
- press top of bottom foot into floor; keep ankle straight
- maintain evenness in hips (resist tendency to shift body to right or left

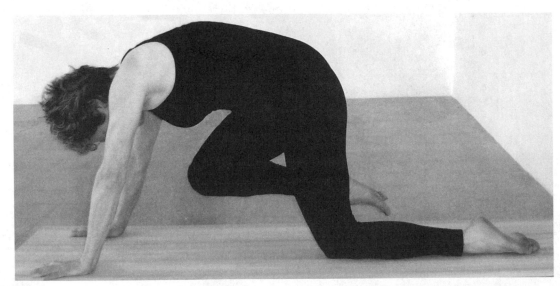

Pointers:

- weight distributes evenly across hands and back to shin or foot
- forearms hug towards each other and backs of shoulders broaden
- neck remains free with jaw relaxed
- thigh comes close to ribs; lower belly flattens

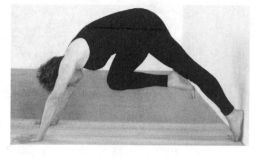

Down Dog Tuck

Back heel and balls of toes press into wall for stability.

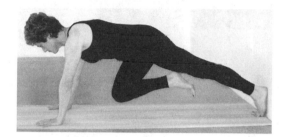

Plank Tuck

Prevent body weight from shifting forward by pressing back heel into wall. back.

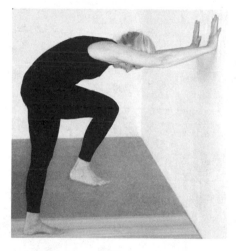

Wall Dog Tuck

Weight evenly distributed across hands; standing foot presses lightly into floor; weight on inner heel and ball of big toe; groins hollow; lower abdomen and quads of raised leg engaged.

PELVIC STABILIZATION CRUNCHES

The following series of dynamic asanas follow nicely from the pelvic and shoulder stabilization work introduced in Chapter 3. In all of them, the trunk is brought towards the legs (flexion). The various leg positions all work to create pelvic stability so that the effort is generated from the abdomen instead of from the lower back. Work with a slow and steady breath rhythm and keep your upper chest wall and heart open and receptive.

Benefits: improves digestion (not only of food but also of emotions); contributes to better posture and integrity of movement and in asana (photos on next page)

Preparation for: almost all other asanas; life

Contraindications: lower back pain and tight psoas

Drishti: tip of nose or up

Wide Angle Crunch

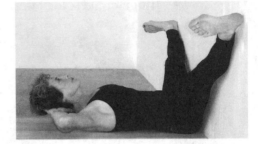

Bound Angle Crunch

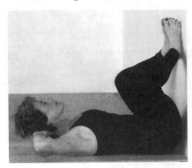

Press outer edges of feet into wall; outer spiral thighs; press head into hands; keep shoulderblades on back.

Press heels into wall and flex toes back; internally rotate thighs and maintain lumbar curve.

Straight-legged Crunch

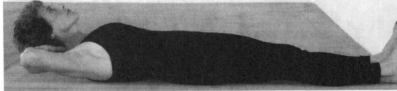

Bent-knee Crunch

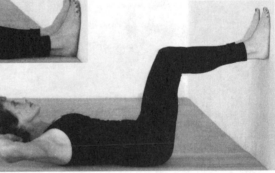

In both, press heels into wall; keep toes active and spread; internally rotate thighs; maintain lumbar curve. Engaging the legs protects the lumbar spine and aids the lift.

Hip-opening Oblique Crunches

Stabilize pelvis by pressing foot into wall and using abdominals and psoas to lower raised hip. Press foot of bent leg into opposite thigh so that there is balanced effort in the legs; hand can lightly press knee.

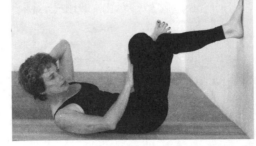

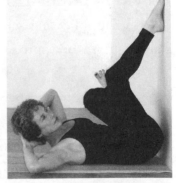

124

Chapter 5

The Architecture Of Practice

Begin with the end in mind.

Stephen R. Covey

5

In structuring an asana session—either for ourselves or for others—it's helpful to know what we're trying to accomplish. Although once attained, yoga is goal-less, getting there, i.e. practice, is not. Whether we merely want to "chill" for a while, bring some relief to a chronically cranky hip, or merge with the divine consciousness inside of all that is, we come to our mats with some intention in mind. Our teachers also have an intent for us. It might be working all the major joints or muscle groups in the body, opening the shoulders in preparation for handstand, or cultivating a deep sense of equanimity. Whatever it is, the intent becomes a blueprint from which the session unfolds.

Say, for example, we wish to create a class that affords full body opening. In such, we would make sure that the spine moves in each of its 6 directions, that the hips flex and extend, ab- and adduct, and rotate both in and out. We would further attend to the abdominal muscles and the lower back through poses that invigorate these tissues. And we would take the shoulders and their blades through their respective and combined paces.

If our intent is to focus on a specific region of the body—for its own sake or in preparation for some more advanced work at a later time—we practice a series of postures that opens the region incrementally. In this case, a well-designed class not only takes a targeted joint through its range of motion, but it also works the muscles in such a way that they're fatigued just enough to let go but not so much that they can no longer function. Muscles are engaged for a given period of time; then they rest. While they do so, the focus of practice shifts to another portion of the body—either to directly counter the effects of the first series of postures or to condition tissues that are related to but not directly involved in the actions that came before.

To effectively address either the full body or a specific portion of it, sequences may be comprised of either dynamic or held postures or a combination of the two. The choice of which to use seems to be a matter of temperament—both for the teacher and the student. While some bodies respond more readily to one method or the other, there is no right or wrong when it comes to deciding whether to be still or to move. There is, to be sure, a difference in result. Held poses tend to foster joint stability; whereas movement fosters mobility. Both cultivate stamina. Proponents of dynamic poses are fond of saying that movement builds fluidity. Those who favor held poses contend that subtlety of awareness is better served when one is still. Both are correct. . .as far as their own experience goes.

126

What follows in this section is a series of potential classes. Two address the body as a whole. The first of these is a very beginning level class suitable for seniors, those new to yoga and the physically challenged. The second is more advanced but works well with beginning students. The third through fifth sequences are mixed level classes designed to cultivate the ability to do specific complex poses—half moon, warrior 3, and handstand.

When I first began teaching at the wall, it was difficult to see how one pose might link to another or how, with a prop so unmoving as the wall, poses could transition gracefully one to another. Gradually, I began to see similarities between the shapes the body takes within certain poses, and I learned to build on these. I also discovered that it was possible to bring movement into some of the poses, which facilitates greater opening for some students. Eventually I came to understand that halting movement and awkward transitions are not an essential components of working at the wall. Most of the sequences that follow have rhythm and fluidity. And, in varying degrees, they all utilize both held and dynamic poses. They demonstrate that, even when up against a wall, we can learn to flow.

Note that the numbers are inconsistent: that is, in some sequences, the breath and repetition counts are odd numbered and in others they follow an even-numbered pattern. This accords with the intent of the sequence. Generally speaking, we think of odd numbers as active, yang, masculine. Even numbers are receptive, yin, feminine. High energy sequences, therefore, utilize 3, 5, 7 and 10 (twice 5); conversely, meditative flows work with 2,4, 6, and 10 breaths and repetitions. In all cases, however, breath counts are approximate and can be varied to suit your needs. In addition, since the duration of a breath is a highly individual event, the breath counts and the amount of time that each sequence takes is approximate.

Full Body Sequences

GENTLE OPENING   A 60-minute sequence for seniors and those new to yoga.

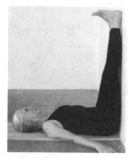 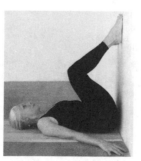 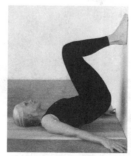 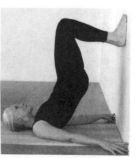

hold 6 breaths   do not hold   inhale & lift; exhale & lower 6-10 times

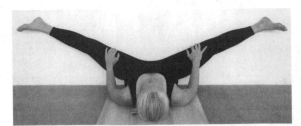
30-60 seconds 30-60 seconds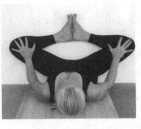

30-60 seconds each side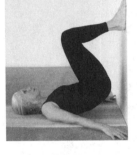

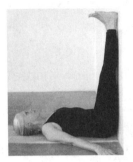 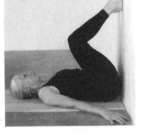 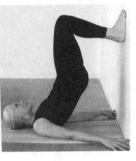

do not hold lift on inhale; lower on exhale 6-10 times

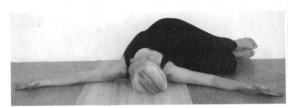

hold each side 8-10 breaths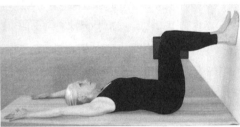

squeeze knees gently and release
8-10 times

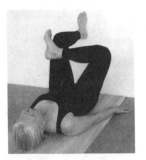 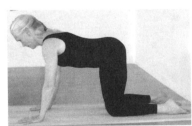 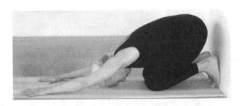

30-60 seconds each side 4 breaths 6-10 breaths

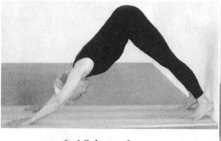
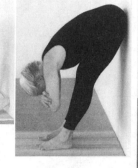
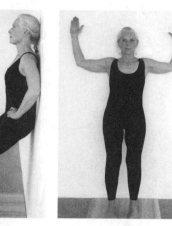

6-10 breaths

6 breaths

6-10 breaths each pose

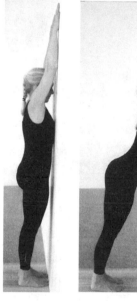
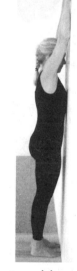
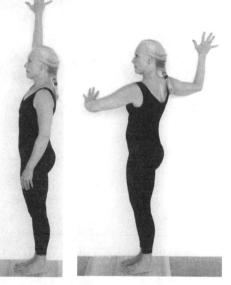

6 breaths each

transition
no hold

6 breaths each pose, turn to
face wall (transition pose),
switch sides

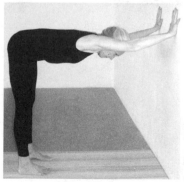
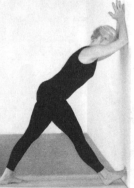
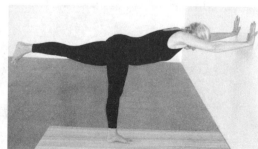

6 breaths

6 breaths, move to next pose, hold 6 breaths, back to
wall dog and THEN switch sides

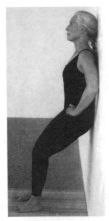

6 breaths

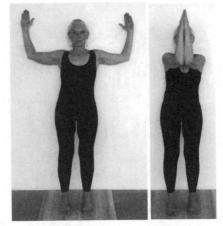

inhale arms open; exhale
arms closed: 6-10 times

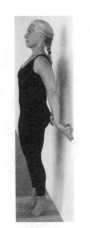

6 breaths

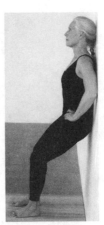

6 breaths

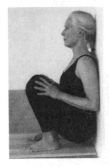

6 breaths

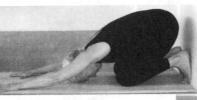

6 breaths

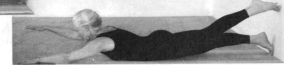

alternate arms and legs; inhale
lift and exhale lower: 6-10 times

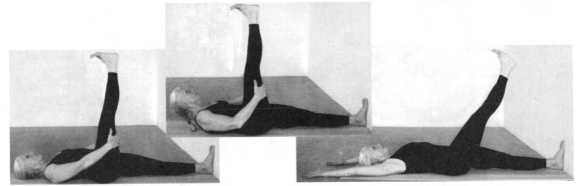

10 breaths hamstring stretch and head lift

exhale as leg lowers

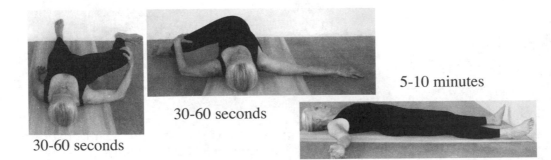

30-60 seconds

30-60 seconds

5-10 minutes

130

CHANGING THE SCRIPT A 75- minute advanced beginners's session that begins and ends with a brief awareness excercise. Static poses are held for 6-10 breaths and dynamic postures are repeated 6-10 times unless otherwise noted.

Take a comfortable seat, facing the wall. Close your eyes and settle into your body. Deepen your breath and encourage even respiration—inhales and exhales equal in length. Notice your sensations and your thoughts. Imagine the wall is a movie screen and your mind a projector. Observe the images you're projecting on the screen in front of you. Breathe steadily 3-4 more times.   Roll to your back; place your feet on the wall so that your ankles are over your knees.

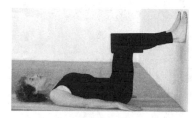
squeeze on exhale; release on inhale

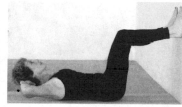
exhale & lift; inhale back

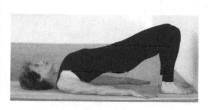
hold

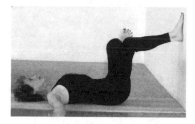
hold and then do next pose

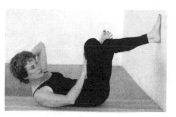
exhale & lift; inhale back

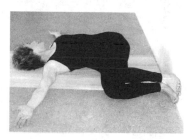
twist to right, hold; then change sides

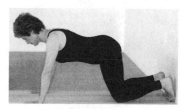
hold

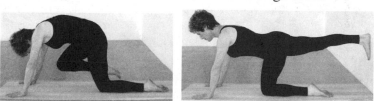
exhale, tuck; inhale, extend; go direcctly to next pose

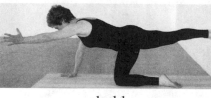
hold

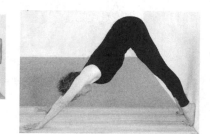

hold down dog; then repeat tuck and extend and balance on other side; finish with a held down dog

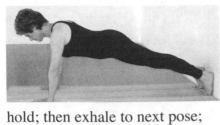

hold; then exhale to next pose; do not hold; inhale back; repeat 2 x

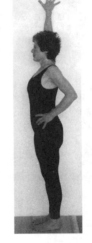

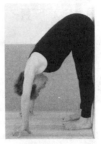

hold

hold each pose in this row; do the arm raise and stretch in sequence on the same side; move to heart opening; then switch sides and go back to heart opening

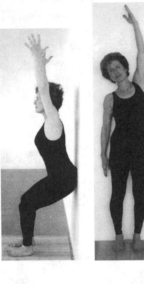

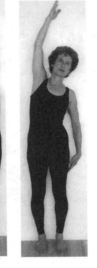

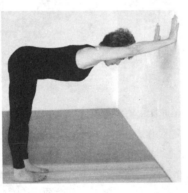

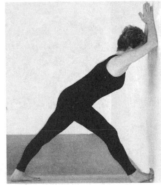

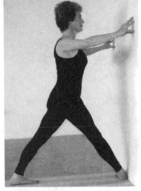

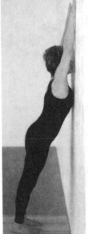

from wall dog, do all poses on the same side, holding each; use wall dog as a transition between sides

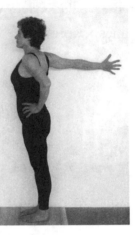

errata: left foot needs to be forward for transition

hold 3 breaths between and after sides

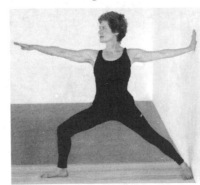

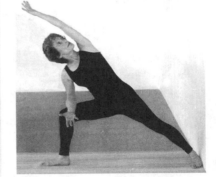

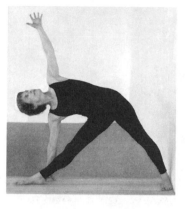 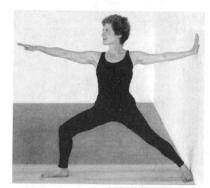 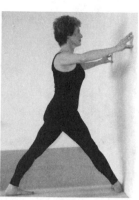

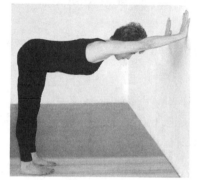

hold wall dog and repeat sequence from calf stretch through wall dog

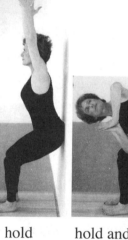

hold   hold and switch
              sides

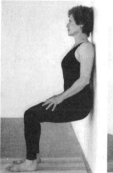 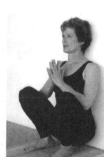 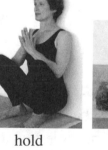 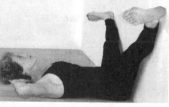

hold   hold   hold   hold

hold each of these 3 poses for at least 60 seconds

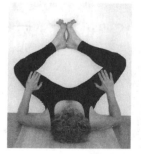 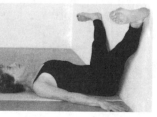 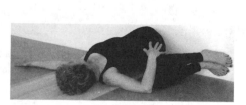

133

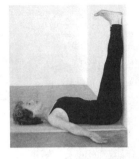 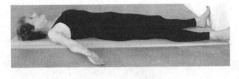

hold either for a minimum of 5 minutes

After complete rest, again sit facing the wall. Breathe deeply and evenly, note your sensations and notice your thoughts. What film is being projected towards the wall in front of you now, and how is it different from the one that you witnessed at the beginning of class?

Stepping Stones to Complexity: Pose-specific Sequences

In the following sessions, the sequencing utilizes a principle called v*inyasa krama*. In this context, *vinyasa* means "to place carefully" and *krama* is a step along the way. *Vinyasa krama*, then, is a sequence that cultivates openness and stability, strength and flexibility in stages, utilizing similarities of shape and action within poses. It also employs muscular and neural patterning in a variety of similar but slightly different (and often more challenging) body positions to condition the nervous system sequentially in order to teach it to accommodate complexity and change. The practices are goal oriented in that they work towards a specific pose, focusing on the joints that will need to be open and the muscles that will be recruited in the chosen asana. The sequences vary in length and difficulty. Modifications for some of the poses in each sequence can be found in Chapter 4.

LIFTING OFF: HALF MOON This 60 minute sequence is one of my favorites because it leads to an effortless half moon, which makes me feel as though gravity is no longer relevant. Prep work begins with pelvic tilting to bring alignment and awareness to the lumbar spine and sacrum because these are key to keeping the lower back, hips, and standing leg comfortable in this one-legged balance pose known in Sanskrit as *ardha chandrasana*. The flow is sutiable for beginning students because the wall assists balance and teaches the role of the back foot as well as the necessity to stack the hips. It begins with core work because the lower abdominals and inner thighs are essential to keeping the body integrated. *Note: unless otherwise specified, all poses are held for 5-7 breaths; dynamic poses use 5-7 repetitions.*

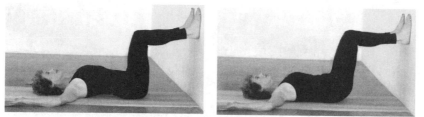

arch lower back on inhale; tuck tailbone up on exhale

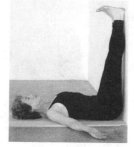

hold

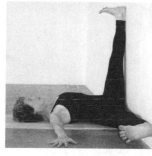 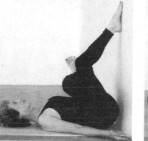

exhale to lift; hold

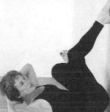 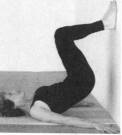

exhale & lift; inhale & lower

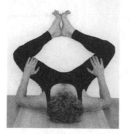 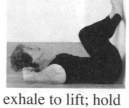

do this row in
sequence and
then switch
sides

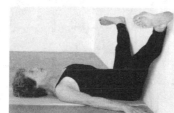 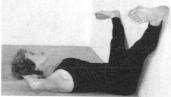

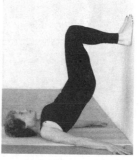

active legs   exhale to lift; hold   hold the lift

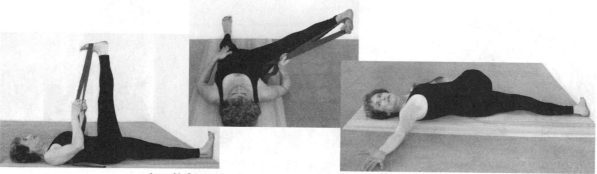

do all 3 poses in sequence before changing sides

135

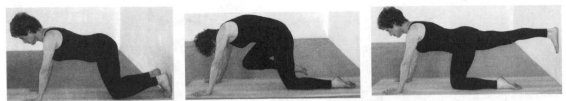

exhale & tuck; inhale & extend; hold foot at wall; then continue with sequence

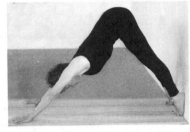

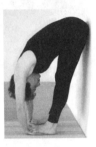

errata: left knee should be down and pose reversed

do tuck and extend, kneeling half moon and down dog in sequence before changing sides

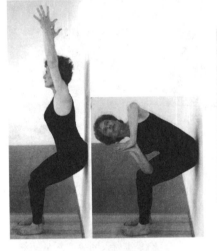

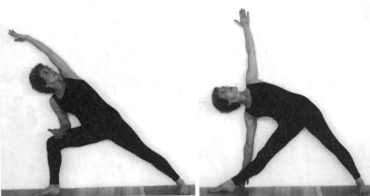

do each of these on same side before switching

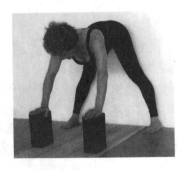

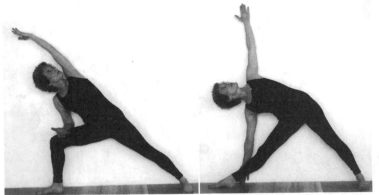

repeat both on both sides

136

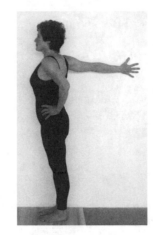
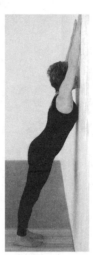

do heart opening
between sides

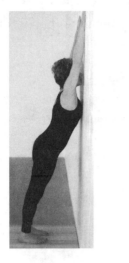

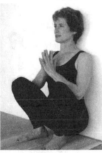

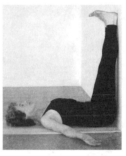

do each side 2x

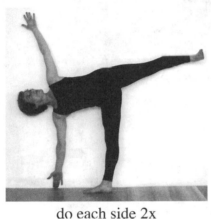

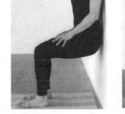

minimum of 5 minutes

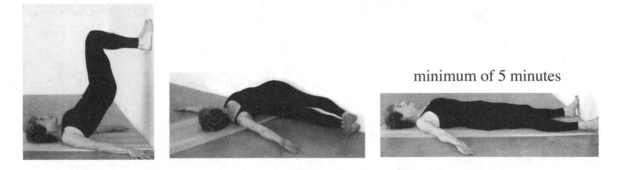

STRAIGHT ARROW: WARRIOR III is a complex pose that requires pelvic stability and core awareness. When done at the wall with a partner assist, it's a marvelous stretch that gently tractions the spine to open and align. *Note: the following 60-75 minute sequence begins with poses that are held just long enough to create a blue print for the movement that immmediately follows as a brief warm up.*

137

Begin by lying on your back, knees straight, feet lightly pressing into the wall. Breath deeply and evenly, feeling your entire body beginning to come alive and your mind becoming sharp and centered.

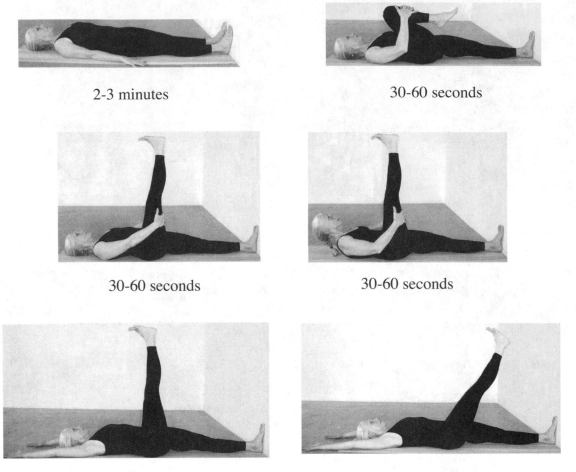

2-3 minutes   30-60 seconds

30-60 seconds   30-60 seconds

30-60 seconds   30-60 seconds

Do each of the last 5 poses on the right in sequences before changing sides. Once the left side is finished, introduce movement as follows: exhale knee in, inhale leg up, exhale head lifts, inhale head and arms back, exhale lower leg and simultaneously draw other leg in. Repeat sequence 5-10 times on each leg.

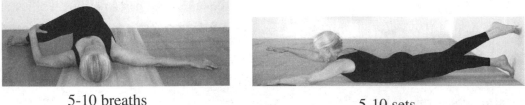

5-10 breaths   5-10 sets

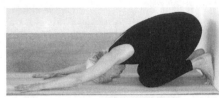

5-10 breaths

do the next 5 poses on the right,
down dog, then do the left side

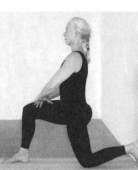

5 breaths

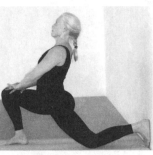

5 breaths

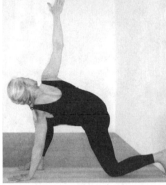

5 breaths

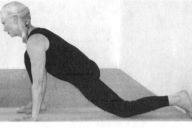

5 breaths

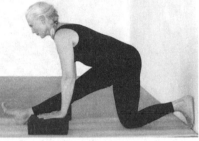

5 breaths

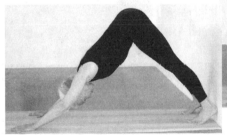

5 breaths

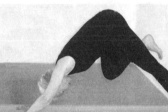

5 breaths each then swittch
sides

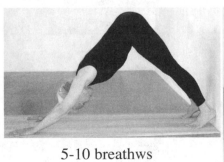

5-10 breathws

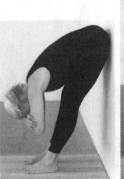

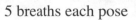

5 breaths each pose

139

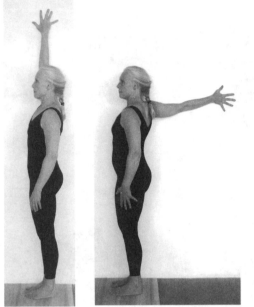 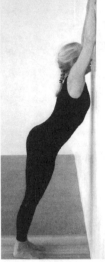 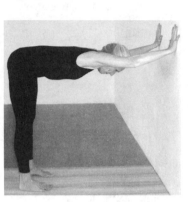

no hold   5 breaths; do heart opening   3 breaths   5-10 breaths
between sides

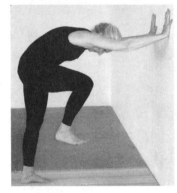 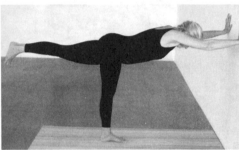 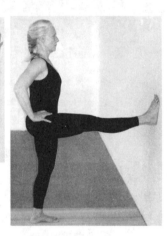

5 breaths each pose on right leg
in sequence; then wall dog and
switch to left side

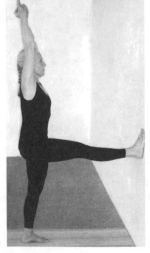 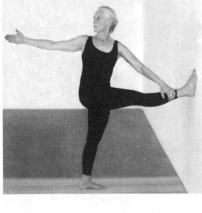 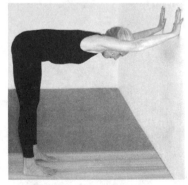

3-5 breaths between
sides and after left

140

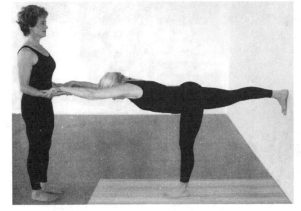
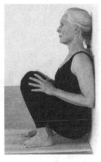

5 breaths each

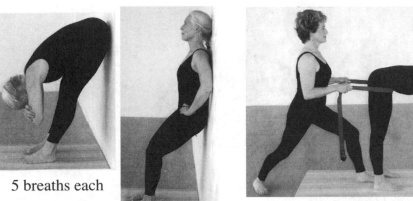

5-10 breaths each partner

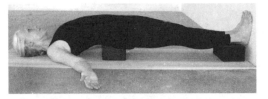

5-10 breaths each side/partner

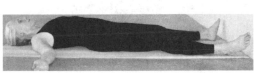

5 breaths

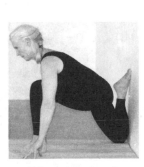

5 breaths each side

may be substituted for sivasana
or used in sequence before it

minimum of 5 minutes

BOTTOMS UP: L HANDSTAND The paradox is that handstand both cultivates and requires openness in the shoulder girdle. The following 60-minute sequence works toward L handstand at the wall, a mighty core and upper body strengthener and a mighty fine shoulder opener. As in the previous session, the amount of time it takes to complete the poses will vary considerably depending on how much energy you have on any day, how quickly or slowly you breathe, and how familiar your body is with the postures.

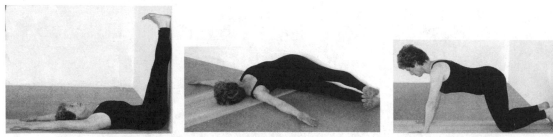

1-3 minutes   1 min. each side   do not hold

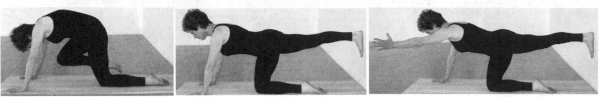

exhale, tuck; inhale extend 3-5 times   5-7 breaths

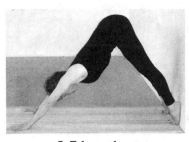 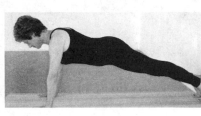 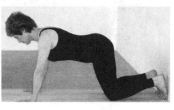

5-7 breaths   5-7 breaths   do not hold

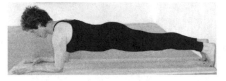 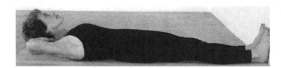

3-7 breaths   hold 5-10 breaths

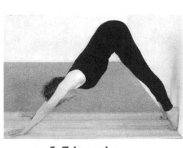 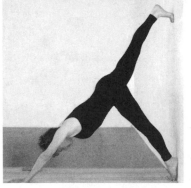 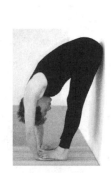

5-7 breaths   5-7 breaths   5 breaths

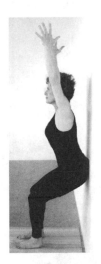

all poses on this page,
5-7 breaths

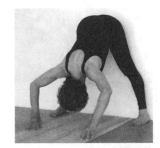

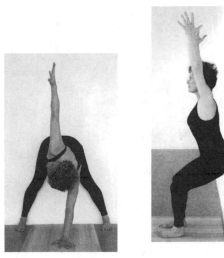

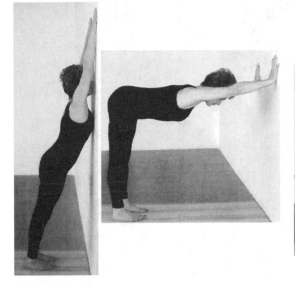

complete the following sequence of 6 poses;
come back to wall dog; then switch sides

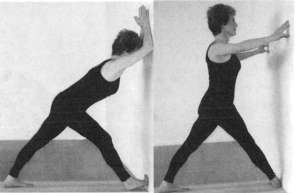

*errata: to make the transition properly the
left foot should be forward in these 2 photos*

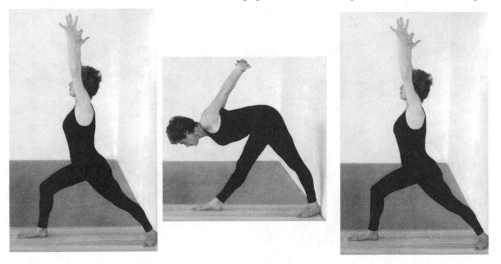

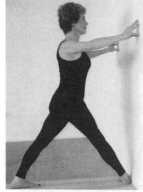 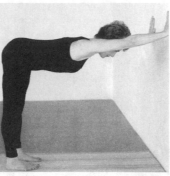 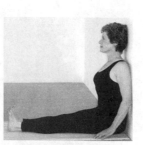

do not hold 2nd time

5 breaths and repeat
sequence on other side

5-10 breaths

5 breaths

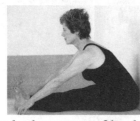 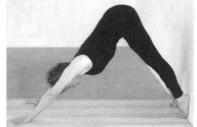 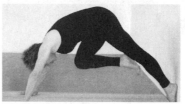

mark placement of heels;
place hands this distance
from wall

do not hold

tuck and reach foot to
wall placing toes on wall
3" above sitz bones

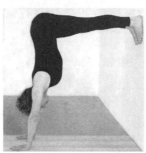 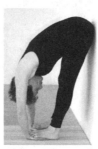 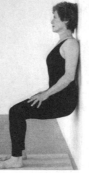 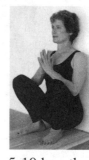

press toes into wall;
bring other foot to wall
and hips over shoulders

5 breaths and
repeat
L handstand

5-7 breaths

5-10 breaths
for this and
next 3 poses

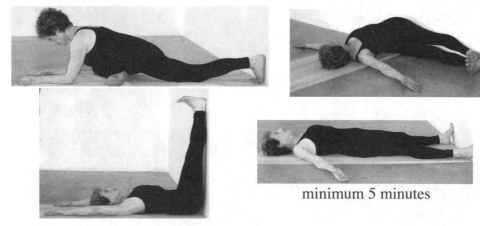

minimum 5 minutes

144

The times for sivasana are given as "at least 5 mintues." This accords with the customary period in many of the classes in metro-Detroit, where I teach. The busy-ness of daily urban-surban life has given rise to classes that are 60-75 minutes long. Students say that they don't have time for longer sessions because of the demands of work, family, and so on. Indeed, although 90 minutes was the usual length of classes when I began to practice, those that are scheduled for more than 75--on the whole--are not well-attended in my area. With the shortening of class time, the duration of sivasana has also been reduced. This has been a huge disservice to students. At 5 minutes, the nervous system is only just beginning to let go; at 10 minutes, a profound shift can be felt in which muscular tension drops away; at 20 minutes the spirit begins to emerge and one can say s/he has truly rested.

Because many of us are conditioned to think of our asana practice as a "workout," we've lost an appreciation for the benefits of rest. So, my advice to anyone working with this material is "If time is an issue, cut out a posture or two and lengthen your repose beyond the minimum suggested time." You'll be amazed at the difference a few more moments of rest make in your sense of well being.

In addition to advocating a longer sivasana than is indicated, I'd also like to say a few words about sequencing. Numerous books and workshop sessions cover the fine art of putting poses together. In general, the best known of the lineages descended from Krishnamacharya (Iyengar, Anusara, Ashtanga, Vinyasa) emphasize the standing poses as templates for training the body in the ways of asana. Tadasana, the warrior I and II families, uttanasana and utkatasana all develop stability and groundedness. They develop the pelvis, legs, and feet and teach us to anchor to the earth in order to gain freedom and openness in the upper body and in the mind and heart.

Other traditions, most notably that of Sivananda and Kundalini yogas begin sessions from different points of departure. In a Sivananda class, head and shoulder stands come early in the practice--without regard for "warming up" the body. The philosphy here is that it's important to awaken the energy centers nearest to the Divine before developing those parts of the body that are most closely in touch with the earth and with our daily lives. Kundalini sessions sometimes loosen and strengthen various muscle tissues at the beginning of each session as needed for whatever energetic sequence is being taught. However, the method does not intend to develop a sequential unfolding of awaress throughout the muscles and bones. Instead the practice aims to directly affect the nervous system and internal organs--and to do so quickly and efficiently.

The point in mentioning other traditions is to encourage experimentation. Within Krishnamcharya's lineage, it's generally accepted that we begin with forward bending and with standing poses because these are the activities that are most familiar to us and to our bodies. Floor poses come after we've developed a measure of communication with the pelvis, feet, and legs. Backbending follows once forward bending has calmed the body and made the spine relatively limber. This is the tradition. However, as with all traditions, there is nothing inherently sacred about it.

The sequences that are included in this chapter more or less adhere to the template. However, they all begin on the floor. In my own practice, floor work often prepares my body for the standing poses. In addition, after a tiring day at work or at the beginning of a lazy Sunday morning, working on the floor serves to make my students ready for the more intense efforts required by the standing postures. In addition, I find that students with lower back issues or a dicey sacrum benefit from backbending placed early in the session.

There is a commonly accepted understanding that yoga is an experiential science and as such, it's exploratory rather than prescriptive. That is to say that we all possess an inner guide who is quite as brilliant as the one who leads our favorite class or the master teacher who has written this or any other book on the subject. What is required is that we learn to be still enough to hear the inner voice.

Of course it's far easier to show up for class and give ourselves over to another's direction for an hour. And in the beginning it may be far more effective to do so and to read books and articles and to learn from the adept. After all, why re-invent the wheel?

At some point, however, we need to be able to run everything past our inner intuitive heart and to say, "Well, that may be the tradition, but it doesn't work for me." In order to live meaningful lives, we need to be able to do this both on and off the mat. We must develop trust in our own ability to discern what's good for us without relying on external guidance. We need to have the freedom to do an intense backbend before doing any forward bending or to hold down dog or triangle or head stand for 5 minutes before we do any warm ups (sun salutations, lunges, cat-cows). Most of all, we need to be increasingly aware of and honor the guru within.

How do we know when the inner voice is that of the persistant 2-year old or s/he who dispels the darkness? How do we know what works and what doesn't? We experiment. We do what we're told, and we do what we're not told and we do what we're told *not* to do (but mindfully and with full awareness of breath and bodily sensations).

So, if your body feels like opening a session with a back bend, do it--but carefully. If you feel like constructing an entire session without once coming to your feet, by all means do so. If you choose to concentrate on standing poses to the exclusion of anything else or you wish to focus on twisting or on abdominal strengtheners, have at it. There are only 3

146

requirements. The first is that you work within the framework of your breath by establishing a deep, meditative rhythm--one that drops you into your body so that you pay attention to what you're feeling and where within each posture (or life situation). The second is that you pay attention to what you're feeling and how you're breathing as you move into and out of and hold postions (and life situations). The third is that you notice your breath and any changes in it as you progress through your practice (and your life). You've probably noticed that all 3 requirements are slightly different phrasings of the same concept: breath and attention are the keys to learning to hear the voice of the inner teacher. The inner teacher, in turn, is s/he who notes effects and consequences and thereby formulates personal rules of thumb for practice (and living).

You may also have noticed--as you looked through the asanas and the sequences that followed them--that many poses are similarly shaped.   In warrior III, for example, the trunk, head, arms and lifted leg form a "T" with the standing leg. This same shape occurs in the variation of supta padangusthasana (supine hand to foot pose) wherein one leg is perpendicular to the floor, the other leg reaches to the wall, and the arms extend beyond the head.   The body also forms a "T" in the variation of standing padangusthasana with one foot at the wall (level with the hips) and the arms raised above the head. And finally, in the version of adho mukha svanasana (down dog) in which a leg is lifted and the foot presses the wall, a "T" is also formed. Because the body's relationship with gravity is different in each of these poses, the actions, that is the ways in which the muscles engage, are also different for each asana. Nonetheless, because the relationships between the limbs and torso are identical, the nervous system can learn about each pose from each of the others.

The caveat for teaching--either ourselves or our students--is that we can use all of the poses to teach all of the poses. In other words, we can think of supta padangusthasan with the arms back and a leg up as a supine warrior III. Of course it's a lot easier to hold one leg aloft than it is to balance the entire body on 1 leg.   But, on our backs, we eliminate the fear of falling that's engendered by attempting to hold ourselves upright on the tiny surface of one foot while the body and arms career forward.   In this non-threatening environment, our muscles and nervous systems can begin to understand relationships, cultivate rudiments of core awareness and experience the integration necessary for balance once the leg and postural muscles are strong and open enough to support the combined weight of the torso and limbs.

Among the benefits of using the similarity between shapes of poses is that effort in a particular direction is reinforced each time a shape is repeated, regardless of the actions involved. This creates a learning that is at once sequential and holistic. Each time we stretch the hamstrings--whether it be lying on our backs with 1 leg raised, standing on 1 foot with the other on the wall, bending forward in down dog with 1 foot pressing into the hard surface behind us, we're reiterating the lesson. It might be drawing the femur into the hip socket while pressing through the ball of the big toe to create leverage. Or it might be using the core to square the pelvis. Perhaps it's both. Regardless, each time we do the actions, the body understands them more, and we increase the effectiveness of our communication with whatever tissues are involved.

If repetition is important for learning the actions of poses, it's no less so for understanding how to make a smooth transition from one posture to the next. And again, this is as true in life as it is on the mat. On the mat our bodies take the shape of the asanas. In our lives, our psyches take the shape of our moods and emotions. We get attitude; we posture. Moving smoothly from one emotional state to the next without being pulled off center is the practice of witnessing that we cultivate on the mat. We note how one asana leads seemlessly to the next and, eventually, we come to understand that--as long as we're fully present in the moment--the events of our lives lead seamlessly one to the next.

At the wall we make transitions by observing anchor points within the framework of each asana and moving from and/or between these fixed points. Thus we can move from child's pose with our heels at the wall to down dog with our heels at the wall, to wall splits (a heel at the wall and the other foot pressing the wall above the hips), to L handstand at the wall (now hands are the anchor points) with relative ease. When a foot is at the wall as in the calf stretch, it's easy to pivot that foot so that the outside edge or the heel is against the wall instead of the toes and then to turn the rest of the body toward the center of the room. Thus we turn from facing the wall to facing the center of the room, setting the body up for any of the warriors or their derivatives. To move to the other side, we merely reverse the pivot and our bodies. Once we become familiar with the concept of using an anchor point to ease ourselves into the next posture, moving fluidly at the wall becomes a piece of cake.

It must be noted, however, that there is nothing holy about making smooth transitions during asana practice. Working first one side and then the other in the same pose before going on to the next makes a lot of sense anatomically as it aims toward balanced opening and symmetry of expression. In additon, flowing among several poses on one side before making a transition by linking postures through their anchor points may dictate differential treatment on each side even though it appeals to one's sense of aesthetics. Again, work out what's best for you (or for your students). Mix and match the sequences and the poses following your own inner direction.

In life, however, I'd like to suggest that smooth transitions make life easier. When we need to change a job or a relationship or a residence, it's important to be able to know

148

what's necessary for our emotional equilibrium and what must be transformed so that we can grow. As Buddhism teachers us, there is nothing that is not changing. Understanding how to be comfortable with change is important to our sense of well being. Anchor points impart a measure of continuity as we shift direction so that our lives can take new shape.

Making transitions is a lesson in skilled grace that many of us could well learn to welcome into our lives. In all of our transitions--both on and off the mat--discernment is the key. We need to know what the anchor is and how to use it--with steadiness, with gratitude, and with a playful attitude. Therein lie our posture and our flow.

Chapter 6

Bringing It All Back Home

Life is what happens while you're busy making other plans.

John Lennon

6

Zeno of Elea was a philosopher and mathematician who lived around the time of the historical Buddha and well before Patanjali is said to have penned the Sutras. This pre-Socratic Greek's contributions to philosophy, recorded in Aristotle's Physics, are called Zeno's Paradoxes One version of one of eight remaining paradoxes goes something like this. If everything at rest occupies a particular space, and if that which is in motion occupies such a space at any given moment, then a flying arrow (or a person walking) is therefore motionless.

The reasoning behind this seeming bit of nonsense is as follows. Moving from point A to point B is an impossible undertaking because within the trajectory that joins these locations there are an infinite number of points that must first be reached. The original span might be cut in half, say, with an interim destination being the halfway point. But this distance can itself be halved and the result further halved and then that result halved again and so on. Halving continues indefinitely; as a result, we get lost in the middle and never reach the end.

The paradox is a bit silly from a practical point of view. Eventually, the distances between points will be so minute that we're able to stand on a slew of them with one foot. And, of course, an arrow in flight does in fact reach a destination. However, if we use Zeno's Paradox as a metaphor for the way we get things done, it has some merit. Many of us have set out to find some information on the internet and become distracted by our e-mail or by YouTube. And many of us have set out from the kitchen to put something away and gotten caught up in tidying the bed or the bathroom because, on the way to returning the object, our attention was derailed. All too many times we've begun a project at work or at home only to find that we don't have the right tools or enough information or the "powers that be" have decided we ought to be doing something else instead. Being distracted--getting stuck in the spaces between point A and point B--is a pretty common occurrence.

Yet things get done. We routinely set goals and work incrementally to realize them. We build a house, working from blueprints through setting the foundation, framing the walls, and finishing the interior. On the yoga mat, we work consistently to open our hips, to gain strength, to become more flexible. We also work on the mat to cultivate focus--the ability to stay the course, to walk or ride or fly from start to finish without getting bogged down in the infinite number of possibilities between the two. Concentration and focus are some of the primary benefits of a consistent yoga practice. So is an appreciation of the journey--the spaces between points that open up to infinity.

For many of us, focus borders on obsession. It becomes a wall against distractions, which is not in and of itself a bad thing. This barrier insulates us from that which is outside the parameters of our agenda; it keeps us on task. Tightly held, it precludes interruptions as well as contact with anything or anybody that might be perceived as a delay or deterrence. For sure, getting sucked into a relative's drama or a related but non-essential project is counterproductive. But so is shutting out a sunrise or a daughter's basketball game because we're too busy. When we focus solely on where we want to be in 10 years or how we want our lives to change or what the finished project will look like, we miss a lot. In this case, Zeno's Paradox is a reminder that the journey, too, is the destination. Instead of thinking that a friends' dinner party or a night at the movies is just one more of an infinite number of distractions between ourselves and where we want to be, yoga helps us understand that focus need not be hard edged or exclusive. Rather, concentration can be softly held; we can be simultaneously one-pointed and open.

Initially, it's the breath that sustains this paradox. We focus on our breathing and allow it to open awareness to the field of equanimity within us. From this still place, we direct our attention to the stuck places we find in body or mind. The breath takes us to witness consciousness, a place from which we can simultaneously experience and observe our lives. This fusion of consciousness with sensation is the hallmark of yoga. It's what allows us to focus without closing ourselves off from that which surrounds us. The subconscious mind is forever plugged into its surroundings. It's only the conscious mind, the mind that says "I want" and "I will" that is shut off from experience.

When we allow our willfulness to solidify, we miss the journey--that is, the spaces in between where we are and where we want to be--the place our subconscious knows instinctively. In contrast, when we cultivate the witness, first on the mat and then in our lives, we learn that focus comes of its own accord. We understand that the walls we build to protect our direction often come from insecurity, anxiety, and fear. Sometimes we're unsure about our abilities; sometimes we're anxious about livelihood or the stability of external conditions on which a goal depends; and sometimes we're terrified that if we stop long enough to let others in, we'll be vulnerable or enjoying ourselves so much we won't want to finish what we started.

Regardless of the reasons, walling ourselves into the cocoon of "getting somewhere" creates stress which often leads to illness and then greater stress because the destination becomes ever more distant. Opening to the between places and allowing ourselves the luxury of getting lost in an appreciation of the moments along the way relaxes us and gives us renewed energy for getting on with what we need or want to do.

A friend of mine tells a story about a favorite yoga teacher. In a particularly hard class,

152

she said "If you're in pain in this pose, take a minute and ask yourself: 'Why?'."

"Why" is the operative question. When we find ourselves in physical or emotional pain, knowing why it's happening helps us alleviate it. When we notice that we're walling ourselves off from people and things, we often need to understand why we're becoming so rigid before we can begin to soften. Witness consciousness leads to the marriage of effort and ease mentioned by Patanjali in the Sutras. Through self observation we begin to see that we do standing poses with our neck and shoulders instead of allowing our legs to do the work they're designed to do. Through self observation we also begin to sense when we're too rigidly adhering to our personal agenda and when we're spending too much time smelling the roses. We learn to sense our internal walls when they first begin to form, and we learn to focus without becoming hard.

Walls contain us, and they support us. They help us align, and they offer resistance when needed. A focused mind and an open heart are the by-products of the marriage of effort and ease within asana. They're also the by-products of working with the breath to recognize and let go of the walls that are no longer useful.

Sthira and sukha--firm and soft, steady and sweet: these describe the body-mind on yoga. We practice at the walls within and outside of ourselves, and we become both stronger and more yielding. Simultaneously we learn to go the distance *and* appreciate the journey.

Acknowledgments

To reiterate the words of countless others, "It's not possible to thank everyone whose energy, ideas, and time have contributed to this work." Nonetheless, I would like to acknowledge the following persons.

Daniel Pietroniro and Robert Gagliardo, for turning me on to yoga and meditation. Jonny and Milla Kest for opening the doors to possibility and for ushering me through them. Barbara Nardi for introducing me to the Yoga of Krishnamacharya. Katherine Lucas for providing the support and space to develop my teaching and the class. Linda Makowski for the depth of her mirror. Linda Kay for her hip openers. My students at Beverly Hills Racquet Club and Karma Yoga, whose affection has been pivotal. Cindy Torges for her contributions to the chapter on fundamentals, for her advice and most of all for "being there" throughout the process. Rhoda Medow for providing the perfect work space. Andrew Blackmore for asking me why I wasn't writing. Natalie Donnelon, Allison Ouellette, Michael Zito, Karen Lutz, Mindy Eisenberg, and Susann Spilkin--all have helped with the photography. Beth Szott, Dan Gwinn and Ellena Rollins for their reading and insights, and Hazel Dawkins for her enthusiastic editing. Lynn Medow for sharing her vision, time and resources. Sarah Birkhill for help with publication costs. For the generous use of her gallery space, Susanne Hilberry. Mindy Eisenberg for making the pivotal phone call and Barbara Heller for playing the middle. Doug Elbinger, for teaching me the rudiments of Photoshop. Erin Howarth for cheerfully answering my questions about layout. Debra Darvick for inspiration and the title. Wayne Johnson and Beverly Price for coaching me through the publishing process. Without the sound advice of Denny Fairchild, this book would not have come together. Thanks to him and to Caprice Aerts for her introduction.

I would especially like to express my gratitude for the influences provided me by the following teachers: Jonny Kest, Ana Forrest, Paul Grilley, Jason Crandell, Sara Davidson, Shiva Rea, Eddie Modestini and Nicki Doane.

Last but not least is Kathy Dib--for asking the all-important question: "Is there a book about yoga at the wall?"

154

Index